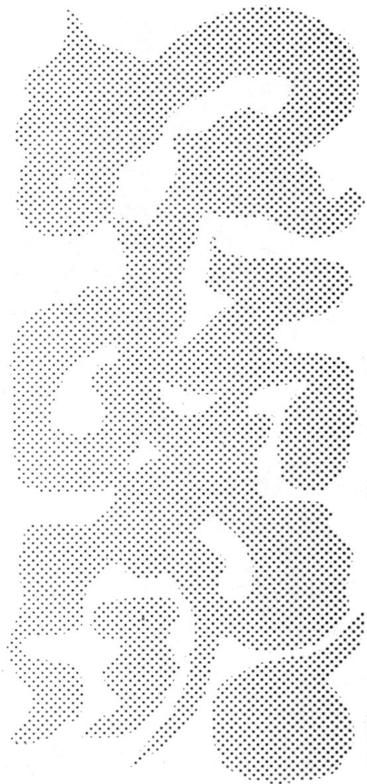

The Daoist talisman on the preceding page represents rising Yang as a positive phenomenon.

Migraines And Traditional Chinese Medicine

A Layperson's Guide

by

Bob Flaws

Blue Poppy Press

PUBLISHED BY:

BLUE POPPY PRESS
1775 LINDEN AVE.
BOULDER, CO 80304

FIRST EDITION
APRIL, 1990

ISBN 0-936185-15-5

Printed at Westview Press, Boulder, CO
Cover printed at D & K Printing, Boulder, CO

TABLE OF CONTENTS

INTRODUCTION

Jane had been working day and night to meet an advertising deadline. The day after the deadline was met, she began a well-earned, two week vacation. In the middle of that morning, she began to feel her fingers become numb and tingly. She also noticed that she could not see clearly. It was as if there was a blank spot in the middle of her visual field. She felt strangely out of sorts, out of synch. Then her head began to hurt on the right side. The pain intensified until it was almost unbearable. Nausea and chills made her misery even worse and any light or noise was unbearable. Drawn up in fetal position in her darkened bedroom, Jane was having a migraine headache. For the next several hours, her agony was intense. Finally, after vomiting, she was able to fall asleep.

Judy gets a migraine every month just before the onset of her period. Like Jane, her headaches are always just on one side. But unlike Jane, Judy's headaches are not linked to any particular lifestyle stresses but rather definitely to her menstrual cycle. Also unlike Jane, Judy does not experience any visual or tactile symptoms before her headaches; nor does she usually get nauseous and vomit. Judy's headaches are more frequent than Jane's, last longer, but are relatively less intense.

Jim, on the other hand, gets clusters of very intense but brief headaches which only last less than an hour. Like Jane, Jim must retreat to a darkened room to ride out the pain which is like a knife in his eye. He may get several such headaches per day for several weeks or even a couple of months. Then he is pain-free for many months or a couple of years. Interestingly, Jim knows when he is about to begin a series of cluster headaches because he gets nosebleeds every day for some time beforehand.

Jane, Judy, and Jim all suffer from some kind of neurovascular or migrainous headache. It is estimated that approximately 10% of men and 20% of women in America and other developed countries suffer from migraine headaches. Although Western medicine offers some help in the treatment of migraines, principally with ergotamine, Inderal, and other such drugs, traditional Chinese medicine treats the full range of neurovascular and migrainous headaches effectively, at low cost, and without drug-induced side-effects. Chinese medicine does this through a combination of acupuncture and herbal therapy supported by diet, exercise, and deep relaxation. In addition, the theory and diagnosis of Chinese medicine vis a vis headaches in general is both enlightening and empowering to its patients in a way Western medicine often is not. Based on traditional Chinese medical theory and diagnosis, headache sufferers can help prevent the occurrence of their headaches through dietary changes, exercise, deep relaxation, and a number of other self-administered, low or no cost therapeutic measures.

Western medicine describes the pain of both migraines and cluster headaches as being due to pressure caused within the head in turn due to vasodilation of the cerebral vasculature. That means the arteries and veins within the skull are jammed full of blood and, therefore, they exert pressure on all the surrounding tissues. This is an accurate physical description. But beyond knowing how mechanically their pain is produced, most sufferers also want to know why this vasodilation occurs in the first place. Unfortunately, further explanations by Western medicine, couched in the terminology of biochemistry, do not really address the issue of why a person gets migraines in terms of human, every day experience. Whereas, the theory of traditional Chinese medicine does.

However, before the theories of Chinese medicine will make sense to a Western layperson, they first need to know a few basic things about the conceptual differences between Western and Chinese medicines. This is because most Westerners are pickled in the ideas and concepts of Western medicine and the material science upon which it is based. Traditional Chinese medicine is based on a different vision of reality, but one which, nevertheless, has stood the test of time. Western medicine seeks to analyze the smallest bits of phenomena it can isolate and only treats as real those things which can be weighed or measured physically or "objectively". The importance of such objective measurements is based on philosophical dualism. That is the view that the world and the mind which perceives the world are two separate entities.

Chinese medicine, on the other hand, is based on a thorough-going holism and non-dualism. That means, from the traditional Chinese medical point of view, there is no duality between the mind and the phenomena it perceives, both of which are co-dependent in their arising. Because of such a non-dualistic philosophical view, Chinese medicine is more interested in functional relationships and patterns of simultaneous arising. Its theories are more general and its truths are derived directly from lived experience. It is often said that Chinese medicine is more interested in energy than matter, and, in one sense, this is true. But even such a statement belies the Western tendency to dichotomize mind and matter, energy and matter, energy and mind. Such dichotomies are not really a part of Chinese medicine's holistic philosophy when it comes to knowing what it knows.

Western laypersons trying to understand the insights and theories of traditional Chinese medicine must, therefore, attempt to see this medicine with a fresh and open mind. The concepts of Chinese medicine have little to do with Western biology and often seem to contradict the nineteenth century biological ideas most of us, including Western physicians, still labor under. However, if the reader can understand that the Chinese concepts of, for instance, the Organs and Bowels are distinct and dissimilar to the Western concepts of the same English names, then one can simply judge the Chinese concepts on their own internal logic and consistency. If we can approach the theories of traditional Chinese medicine with such a fresh and open mind and with as few preconceptions as possible, we will find that Chinese medicine is a remarkably coherent, rational, humane, and wise vision of human experience.

This book is an attempt to present to Western laypersons the traditional Chinese medical theories regarding the cause, diagnosis, and cure of neurovascular headaches. In traditional Chinese medicine, there is no category of neurovascular headache per se. This is a Western medical disease category. However, it is my experience that traditional Chinese medicine can accurately and adequately explain all the various signs, symptoms, and idiosyncracies of neurovascular headaches. Therefore, this explanation of migrainous and neurovascular headaches is, in a sense, a hybridization of Western disease categories explained by the rationale of traditional Chinese theories. As such, I believe it provides an integration of modern experience with age-old wisdom and offers the contemporary migraine sufferer the best of both worlds.

Ironically, the traditional Western medical understanding of migraines up until one hundred years ago was essentially identical to the traditional Chinese understanding. Therefore, paradoxically, Westerners accepting the traditional Chinese medical view of this disease, rather than adopting a foreign and exotic import, are, in a sense, returning to their own philosophical roots.

This book begins first with the Western categorization and description of neurovascular headaches. This is followed by a general description of the cause and diagnosis of headaches in traditional Chinese medicine. Then, based on such understanding, I attempt to explain in Chinese medical terms the reasons for all the various signs, symptoms, and idiosyncracies of migraine. This is followed by a section on the Chinese theory of the prevention of migraines which includes self-administered dietary, exercise, and deep relaxation therapies. Also included are sections on other self-administered, first aid treatments and on the professional treatment of neurovascular headaches with acupuncture and Chinese herbal medicine. In conclusion, I discuss how a potential patient interested in availing themselves of the benefits of traditional Chinese medicine can find a professional practitioner in the United States.

In addition, I have included three appendices. The first is a brief historical review of Western medical theory vis a vis migraines and a comparison with traditional Chinese medical theory. The second appendix is a discussion of the traditional Chinese medical description of the most common Western pharmaceuticals used to treat migrainous headaches. It is my belief that Chinese medical theory can more wisely discriminate the use of such medicinals and explain why they cause the side-effects they do. And the third appendix is a discussion of the psycho-spiritual ramifications and implications of migraine.

Throughout this book, I must, by necessity, continuously speak of traditional Chinese medicine as opposed to modern Western medicine. However, I hope that the reader will come to see by the end of this book that "Chinese medicine" is only the name for a style of thought or a medical philosophy. Ultimately, such a medical philosophy is only valuable to the world at large if its methodology transcends cultural biases and ethnocentric limitations. It is my belief that so-called Chinese medicine has the capability of being a universally valid theory and methodology of medicine and that it both could and should be the basis for the establishment of a truly wise and humane, professional, holistic, planetary medicine for the 21st century.

If this books helps to bring clarity and understanding to Western migraine sufferers and, therefore, helps to alleviate their pain, it will have served its primary purpose. But, if it also helps to bridge the gulf between modern Western and traditional Chinese medicines, it will have also served a higher purpose through which unlimited persons may be benefitted in the future. In any case, this is my hope.

THE WESTERN MEDICAL DESCRIPTION OF MIGRAINES

There are several different types of migraines. Modern Western medicine divides migraines into three distinct groups. These are classical migraines, common migraines, and migrainous neuralgia or cluster headaches. In addition, there are also various subcategories which are described in this chapter. It is also useful to understand the Western concepts of tension headaches, sinus headaches, and brain tumor headaches in order to distinguish these from migraines.

CLASSICAL MIGRAINE

According to Dr. James W. Lance, MD,

> Classical migraine is easily recognized because it is preceded by visual disturbance. This may consist of little specks or flashes of light that appear in front of the eyes, blurred eyesight, or a more complicated pattern of zigzags that moves slowly across the field of vision for twenty or thirty minutes. As this subsides, aching starts in the front or back of the head, usually on one side, and progressively becomes more severe. The victims feel sick and may vomit. Light hurts their eyes; they may retire to a dark room and try to sleep it off.[1]

Based on the above description, we can say then that the definition of a classical migraine is a headache which begins with some sort of visual disturbance, proceeds to one-sided head pain, and which involves nausea and possibly vomiting. Although the pain may begin on one side, as it progresses, it may diffuse to involve the whole head. Unless these three factors are present during a headache episode -- visual disturbance, head pain, and stomach upset -- one does not have a so-called classical migraine. The length of time between successive attacks of classical migraine is usually somewhere between two and ten weeks, individual patients generally adhering fairly closely to their own time patterns.[2]

COMMON MIGRAINE

A common migraine is not preceded by any visual disturbance. There is no particular prodromal warning sign as with classical migraine.

> The headache may come on in the early hours of the morning and awaken the subject, or it may come on at any other time of the day. It usually (but not always) involves only one side of the head and usually (but not always) is accompanied by nausea and aversion to light ... The less frequent and more severe the headache, the more likely it is to have the characteristics of migraine. The more frequent the headache, the more likely it will be of a milder form, involving both sides of the head and not associated with nausea and aversion to light.[3]

As Dr. Lance notes, because there is no definite prodromal visual disturbance, common migraine is more difficult to diagnose conclusively.[4] Most people, when they think of migraine, assume such a headache is one-sided. However, this is not always the case. Dr. J. Olsen of Copenhagen surveyed 678 migraine sufferers and found that

44%	experienced	one-sided, temporal headache
22%	"	headache all over the head
14%	"	bilateral frontal headache
13%	"	one-sided frontal headache
6%	"	occipital headache
1%	"	headaches at their vertex[5]

However, common migraine headaches tend to be, more often than not, one-sided and accompanied by digestive upset. In addition, their pain tends to be more acute at onset and more severe than ordinary tension headaches. Frequent, periodic common migraines tend to occur most often at night.[6]

CLUSTER HEADACHE

Cluster headaches were first described in Western medical literature by Mollendorf in 1867. Since then they have been known by a succession of names depending upon the dominant theory of their mechanism. They have been called ciliary neuralgia, splenopalatine neuralgia, Horton's cephalgia, histamine headaches, and migrainous neuralgia besides cluster headaches. As a species of migraine, they are mechanically due to increased pressure in the veins and arteries of the head. They are called cluster headaches since they occur in clusters or groups.

These clusters generally present one to three times per day for periods of six to twelve weeks at a time. They tend to last less than an hour apiece. They are usually one-sided and centered in or around the eye. The eye on the affected side may become bloodshot or water. Often the eyelid droops and the pupil contracts. Typically, the nostril on the affected side either becomes blocked or runs. Slight nausea is possible as an accompanying symptom as is pronounced photophobia. The scalp over the affected area may feel tender to the touch and little hive-like bumps may be felt inside the mouth.[7] 85% of cluster headache sufferers are men.[8]

Cluster headaches are very much linked to biorhythms. They tend to cycle daily at specific hours and also yearly. Dr. Oliver Sacks, MD, remarks that Easter is the "usual cluster season".[9] According to Dudley and Rowland, the remission period averages twelve months, i.e. one year.[10] Dr. Sacks considers an entire cluster sequence as a form of periodic migraine: "We may also consider cluster headache as a form of periodic migraine, provided that we regard the entire cluster (which may comprise a hundred individual attacks of migrainous neuralgia) as a single monstrous attack of migraine."[11]

Of the above three described types of migraine, common migraine is the most commonly experienced. Next in frequency is classical migraine, and cluster headaches are relatively rare. Whether classical, common, or cluster, migraines can include a huge variety of signs and symptoms. As Dr. Sacks writes,

> Compact and clearly defined at its centre, migraine diffuses outwards until it merges with an immense surrounding field of allied phenomena. The only boundaries which exist are those which we are forced to adopt for nosological clarity and clinical action. We construct such boundaries and limits, for there are none in the subject itself.[12]

A more complete list of the possible signs and symptoms accompanying migraine are: visual disturbances, dizziness, hallucinations, nausea, vomiting, numbness or tingling, sensitivity to light, noise, smell, and/or flavor, depression, irritability, tension, detachment, yawning, hunger, talkativeness, loss of memory for words, names, etc., slurred speech and incoherence, trembling and tremor, pain, skin rash, swelling of the fingers, hands, wrists, ankles, breasts, legs, and/or abdomen, inability to concentrate, constipation, diarrhea, and increased or decreased urination.[13] As Dr. Sacks, my personal favorite Western medical authority on migraine points out, migraine is not just a headache. It is the entire constellation of signs and symptoms experienced within the prodromal aura, the headache itself, and its recovery period.[14]

Other subcategories of migraine include: menstrual migraine, hemiplegic migraine, ophthalmoplegic migraine, facial migraine, basilar migraine, and migraine equivalents.

MENSTRUAL MIGRAINE

Menstrual migraine is the occurrence of migrainous headache in synchronization with the monthly menstrual cycle. Approximately 20% of women suffer occasional premenstrual migraines.[15] However, menstrual migraines are not always premenstrual. They may come after the onset of the period, after it has just finished, or at mid-cycle. They may be either classical or common in form. Such menstrual migraines usually cease with pregnancy and menopause.

HEMIPLEGIC MIGRAINE

This type of migraine is relatively rare. It was first described in the Western literature by Liveing in the mid-nineteenth century.[16] Liveing, in his classic book on migraines, or megrim as he called them, referred to this type of migraine as a kind of apoplectic seizure. Persons suffering from hemiplegic migraines experience, in addition to their other signs and symptoms, one-sided muscular weakness or paralysis and/or one-sided numbness or loss of sensitivity. Usually, these persons are chronic migraineurs and experience such hemiplegia at rare and infrequent intervals. The symptoms of such migrainous hemiplegia usually last several hours to, at worst, a couple of days.

OPHTHALMOPLEGIC MIGRAINE

Similar to the above, ophthalmoplegic migraine is quite rare and occurs in chronic migraineurs. Dr. Sacks reports an incidence of only eight cases of ophthalmoplegic migraine in 5000 cases.[17] Ophthalmoplegia means paralysis of the eye. This is a transient phenomenon which may last several hours of more.

FACIAL MIGRAINE

Facial migraine is characterized by pain which begins in the eye or cheek and may extend to the teeth. Its pain is usually less severe than other forms of migraine but lasts a much longer time.[18] It may be accompanied by photo and/or phonophobia, and it is my experience that it may present in older patients with a previous history of common or classical migraines.

BASILAR MIGRAINE

This rare form of migraine is most often encountered in teenage girls.[19] It gets its name from the fact that its pain is mostly occipital or at the base of the skull. Its accompanying signs and symptoms can include incoherent or slurred speech, giddiness or fainting, and visual disturbance.[20]

MIGRAINE EQUIVALENTS

Migraine equivalents are various periodic complaints which do *not* include headache but which do include other of the prodromal or accompanying signs and symptoms of migraine. Some Western authors use the term migraine equivalent to mean the experience of a migrainous aura but without the subsequent development of headache. In such cases, the person may experience the scintillating specks of light in their vision and the numbness and tingling of their extremities which are common prodromal or premonitory signs of migraine headache. However, they may not ever experience anything further than that.

On the other hand, Dr. Sacks includes a number of other, related disorders under the heading of migraine equivalents. These include cyclic or periodic vomiting and bilious attacks, abdominal migraine, i.e. abdominal pain, periodic diarrhea, and precordial or pseudo-angina migraine.[21] The first three of these are relatively self-explanatory. The last refers to periodic gripping chest pain which mimic angina pectoris and is sometimes mis-diagnosed as that. Dr. Sacks reports seeing only 2 cases of precordial migraine in 1000 migraine cases[22]. So this particular malady is quite rare.

All of these experiences may alternate with periodic migraines on an occasional basis or individuals may only experience one or the other of these forms of migraine equivalents. This clearly shows that migraines are a process and that this process can take various forms depending upon the individual and a host of other contributory factors. In other words, migraines are not a simple, discrete disease, such as strep throat or bacterial dysentery.

Rather, they are a multifaceted and complex aberration of internal functioning. One does not have migraines; one is migrainous. And just as an individual is constantly changing from moment to moment and day to day, and just as each person is unique, so this migrainous process can take a multiplicity of forms.

Therefore, throughout Western medical history, doctors have attempted to define a migrainous personality. Up until the last forty years or so, Western doctors from Galen to Liveing have felt that there is indeed a migrainous personality. The classical Western description of the typical migraineur is a person who is "tense, meticulous, and obsessional in nature."[23] Dr. James Lance also states: "As a general rule, happy people have fewer headaches than sad people..."[24] Such general, clinical impressions, however, have not been supported by recent statistical research and some contemporary authors are vehement in their rejection of a typical migrainous personality. Authors Dudley and Rowland, in *How to Find Relief from Migraine*, state flatly and unequivocally, "There is no such thing as the 'migraine personality'."[25] This underscores the fact that, as we will see below, there are a number of factors which can trigger migraines, personality being only one of these.

Nonetheless, although modern researchers reject the notion of a migraine personality, migraine sufferers are prone to certain other disorders which do, in fact, form a kind of constellation. Migraineurs as a group tend to experience ulcerative colitis, psoriasis, hayfever, asthma, urticaria, Meniere's disease, peptic ulcer, Crohn's disease, nightmares, PMS, constipation, diarrhea,[26] tension headaches, functional heart disease, essential hypertension, rhinitis, upper respiratory tract infections, psychoneuroses, and motion sickness.[27] This is a seemingly diverse list of maladies which one might say anyone might have one or more. However, as we will see further on, according to Chinese medical theory, there are very definite reasons why a person with migraines might also experience these specific other diseases and complaints.

THE NATURAL HISTORY OF MIGRAINES

As a phenomenal event, migraines have a beginning, a middle, and an end. Dr. Sacks divides the course of an individual migraine episode into five stages or phases:

1) Excitation
2) Engorgement
3) Prostration
4) Resolution
5) Rebound

Excitation

The period of excitation refers to the prodromal or aura phase of a migraine in process. It is characterized by changes in mood, hyperacusis or hypersensitivity, visual disturbance, and paresthesia nor numbness and tingling. Dr. Lance estimates that approximately 20% of migraine sufferers experience premonitory symptoms for up to 24 hours before the attack itself.[28]

Typically, the first premonitory signs are changes in mood and levels of arousal. Suffers may feel elated or depressed. They may be angry, irritable, enraged, or aroused. They often experience restless hyperactivity and insomnia. In general, these can all be characterized as excessive subjective states. Such subjective changes in one's sense of self can include states of altered consciousness, such as *deja vu* and *jamias vu*. *Deja vu* is the feeling of having experienced something before. *Jamais vu* is just the opposite. It is a feeling of complete unfamiliarity, strangeness, and disconnection. Some people experience a "doubling of consciousness"[29] and other such states of expanded consciousness.

Sacks describes seven qualities to such prodromal altered states of affect or consciousness:

1) Sudden onset
2) Apparent sourcelessness vis a vis current sensory stimuli
3) An over-whelming or compelling quality

4) Passivity or a feeling of these experiences "forced" into the mind
5) Brief duration
6) A sense of stillness and/or timelessness
7) The impossibility of adequate description

As Sacks goes on to say:

> Such states of overwhelming 'forced' feeling may occur not only in cerebral paroxysms as migraine and epilepsy, but in schizophrenic and drug-induced psychoses, in feverish and toxic states, in hysterical, ecstatic, and dream states. We are inevitably reminded of William James' listing of the qualities of 'mystical' states: ineffability, noetic quality, transciency, passivity.[30]

We will discuss the implications of such altered states in the appendix on the relationship between migraines and spiritual experiences.

Along these same lines, hyperacusis or being more sensitive to sensory stimuli than normal is also common during migrainous auras. This can be hypersensitivity to light, sound, smell, taste, or touch, although hypersensitivity to sound and light are the two most common forms of hyperacuity. Often, hypersensitivity to light is combined with various visual disturbances of which there are a number of kinds identified in the literature. These are generally referred to as scotoma (singular) or scotomata (plural). In their simplest form, they may be sparks of scintillating light. They may also take the form of crenelated or jagged geometric shapes which move across the visual field. These are called fortification spectra. There may be blank spots in the visual field in which the patient cannot see anything. These are called negative scotomata. Or one may see everything very small or very large or as if through a narrow tunnel. Approximately one third of migraineurs experience some kind of visual disturbance lasting, on an average, 20-45 minutes before any pain begins.31

Also, approximately one third of migraineurs experience pins and needles in their hands, face, mouth, or tongue.[32] Technically, this is called paresthesia. Frequently also, migraine sufferers experience increased hunger during their prodromal period and/or water brash. Water brash means one's mouth fills with hypersalivation, often of a sour, acidic taste.

Engorgement

Dr.Sack's period of engorgement corresponds to the initial onset of the pain. It is characterized by muscular tension, visceral distention, vascular dilation (causing pain), constipation, decreased urination, fluid retention, restlessness, irritability, and anxiety.[33] "The patient is restless and agitated; if confined to his bed, he will move about constantly, rearranging the bedclothes, finding no position of comfort; he will tolerate neither sensory nor social intrusions."[34] Although rare, migraineurs at this stage may experience muscular spasms and convulsions. Accounts of such spasticity are found in the Western classical literature on migraines.[35] All these signs and symptoms bespeak an excess of something which has built up and, seemingly, become stuck somehow.

Prostration

Next comes prostration. During this phase, the patient becomes apathetic, depressed, nauseous, drowsy, faint, or stuporous. They experience a general malaise and muscular slackness or weakness. Typically, patients retreat from all stimulation.[36] Some few patients may even become unconscious during this phase. However, when they do, they tend to slide into an unconscious, stuporous state.

> Migraine syncope is never of abrupt onset and offset, like a *petit mal* attack; the patient sinks into it over the course of a few minutes, and regains his faculties in the same gradual fashion. It is convenient to recognize three stages in this context: first a stage of torpor and lethargy; secondly a stage of stupor in which the patient may suffer 'forced' thought and imagery, generally with an unpleasant

quality -- Liveing speaks of 'horrid trances' at this stage ... (and) thirdly, a stage of coma, which is likely to be accompanied by incontinence, and very occasionally, by seizure-activity. In some cases, this stage of prostration may be the end of the attack, there being three clinically recognized ways a migraine may end: exhaustion, crisis, or lysis.[37]

Resolution

The fourth phase in the course of an individual attack is resolution. If the patient does not simply sleep off the attack, it may be brought to an end by crisis. This means that the attack may be terminated by a "sudden accession of physical or mental activity which brings the attack to an end within minutes."[38] This may be occasioned by exercise, sex, or a sudden experience of fright, rage, or other strong emotion. When the attack is resolved by such a crisis, the stages of prostration and resolution may be, in a sense, reversed. The patient may experience crisis followed by recuperative sleep or may pass through a period of passivity.

In the same way, if resolution comes through lysis, either there will not be prostration or sleep will come after such lysis. Lysis means some excretory activity. Typically in the case of migraine, this means vomiting. However, it can also potentially include diarrhea, crying, or even perspiration. In some cases, there is lysis, i.e. vomiting, but this fails to relieve the headache. The person continues to vomit bile and may even have dry heaves accompanied each time by unbearable exacerbation of their headache. Eventually, such persons usually become prostrate and sleep their attack off.

Rebound

Rebound describes the post-attack recovery. After crisis, lysis, or exhaustion, and typically after sleeping, the sufferer experiences renewed energy and a return to their normal mood. In many cases, the person will feel even better than usual, in fact, euphoric. Rebound euphoria or feeling especially well after a migraine attack tends to occur no matter how the attack is resolved, whether through sleep, crisis, or lysis.

PERIODICITY

On the large scale of a person's entire life, migraines tend to begin fairly early. 43% of migraineurs develop their first migraines between the ages of 11 and 20.[39] This means that most people develop migraines at or around puberty. This tendency has been a well established fact since at least the 1870s and Edward Liveing. Many Western authorities also agree that even before the onset of actual migraines at puberty, many migraineurs suffer from recurrent stomachaches and nausea as children. Sacks cites one study of 198 migraine sufferers of whom 31% recalled frequent 'bilious attacks' as children, while 59% had at least one of more bilious attacks and/or severe motion sickness.[40] Some researchers also see infantile eczema as a precursor to the development of a "migrainous constitution".[41]

It is also a fact that migraines tend to get better with age. The exception to this tendency are certain women whose headaches either worsen at menopause or begin with their climacteric.[42] However, in most people migraine attacks tend to get fewer after the age of forty-five.[43] Dr. Wilkinson says the reason for this in Western medicine is not known.

Dr. Lance sums up and reiterates the lifetime trend in the course of migraines:

> Migrainous symptoms may first appear in early childhood and alter in character as the child grows. A child may suffer from vomiting and abdominal pain (bilious attacks) at an early age whenever there is a party or some other excitement. A little later, the child may complain of headache accompanying the vomiting attacks, which recur every few months. At puberty, these episodes may be heralded by shimmering or blurred eyesight or even by spectacular zigzags of color that move slowly across the field of vision, leaving blank spots

behind where vision is impaired or completely lost. The headaches may have a 60 percent chance of disappearing in the late teens but may persist, in which case nausea is often less prominent and vomiting may cease to be a part of the attack. Those children who do lose their headaches in adolescence have about a 30 percent chance of recurrence in later years, so that about 60 percent of migrainous children will still be subject to migraines in their thirties. In middle life, the headaches may cease and the patient may be left with the visual disturbance only, which is then called a migraine equivalent ... Some develop migraine for the first time in their fifties, but it is more common for the migrainous tendency to abate gradually. Affected adults have a 70 percent chance of losing their headache or improving substantially over the course of fifteen years or so.[44]

On the small scale of the time elapsed between attacks, it is possible to identify two types of migraines: periodic and paroxysmal. Periodic migraines seem to be related to biorhythmic cycles irrespective of lifestyle and dietary factors. Periodic migraines tend to occur at certain intervals depending upon the individual's own internal clock. Whereas, paroxysmal migraines are irregularly or widely separated in time and tend to be triggered by certain specific stimuli, such as fatigue, diet, stress, strong emotional reactivity, and weather changes. As mentioned above, the more widely spaced the attack, the more severe it is likely to be.

Dr. Sacks, speaking of periodic migraines, says:

> There is characteristically a time of absolute immunity to further attack following every severe attack of periodic migraine...
>
> The immunity diminishes by degrees, and the likelihood of the next attack increases commensurately. Following the termination of absolute immunity, gross provocation may elicit a

> (somewhat premature) attack. As the relative immunity grows less, more and more trifling stimuli may suffice to detonate the impending attack. Finally, when the attack is 'due' (or a little overdue) it *will* occur, explosively, whether or not there is any provocation.[45]

Also as mentioned above, migraines in women tend to be periodic in relationship to their menstrual cycle. Peter Evans, in *Mastering Your Migraine*, states, "Attacks in women seem to be most frequent in the early days of a period -- and in the week directly after the period ends..."[46] It is also not uncommon to find women who at a certain time in their life have "severe menstrual syndromes for several years, (to) lose these to acquire frequent attacks of paroxysmal headache or abdominal pain unrelated to the menstrual period, finally reverting to the original pattern of menstrual disturbance."[47]

It is also a common pattern for migraine sufferers to experience an attack on the weekends. Again Evans says, "If there is any weekly pattern, there is intensification on the weekends."[48] In my experience, however, this weekend pattern is not so much due to any internal biorhythm as it is to an idiosyncratic reaction to stress, since persons also may experience migraines when they go on vacation or following the release of some stressful situation irrespective of the day of the week or what they are doing at the moment.

Thomas Willis, in *De Anima Brutorum* written in 1672, in discussing the various factors which may give rise to migraines, mentions that "changes in season ... (and) the great aspects of the sun and moon" may give rise to migraine attacks.[49] In some people, migraines may be linked to the phases of the moon, the full moon being a time when many migraineurs suffer an attack. However, depending upon the kind of migraine, some persons may also suffer more attacks at the new moon. In terms of change in season, spring is a time when more migraines tend to occur in many patients.

EPIDEMIOLOGY

Epidemiology means the distribution of a disease within a population. As stated above, more women get migraines than men at a rate of about 2 to 1. Migraine is encountered in all cultures throughout the world. At the present time, it does not seem to be concentrated in any particular economic groups. Many Western authorities believe that there is a hereditary factor in migraines. According to Dr. James W. Lance, migraines usually run in families. 60% of sufferers have a close family member who also has some form of migraines.[50] Rose and Gavel state, "There is no doubt that migraine is a familial disorder."[51] However, that does not mean that migraine is necessarily an inherited or genetic disorder. The tendency for migraines to run in families may be explained either as a genetic predisposition or a learned pattern of behavior.

THE CAUSE OF MIGRAINES

Western medicine says that the cause of migrainous headache pain is due to dilation of the blood vessel in the brain which causes increased pressure on the surrounding tissue. Western medicine then goes on to talk about the neurochemistry that causes this dilation or engorgement. Although such neurochemical events involving serotonin and adrenalin no doubt do occur, such descriptions are not very enlightening nor empowering to the individual migraine sufferer.

However, on the human level, Western medicine does identify certain triggering factors which can precipitate a migraine attack. Rose and Gavel give the following list of triggering factors:

Anxiety, tension, depression, shock, frustration
Exhaustion, exercise, sex
Irregular meals, fasting, alcohol
Smoking
Certain foods
Changes in biological rhythm or sleep/wake patterns
Menstruation, menopause, oral contraceptives
Glare, weather changes, cold

Hot baths
High blood pressure, facial pains
Head colds, hayfever[52]

The first group of trigger factors are mostly emotional. Dr. Sacks considers this group to be *the* most important causative factors.

> *Violent emotions* exceed all other acute circumstances in their capacity to provoke migraine reactions, and in many patients -- especially sufferers from classical migraine -- are responsible for the vast majority of attacks experienced...
>
> We find, in practice, that sudden *rage* is the commonest precipitant, although *fright* (panic) may be equally potent in younger patients. Sudden *elation* (as a moment of triumph or unexpected good fortune) may have the same effect...[53]
>
> Such reactions have a paradoxical quality, in that they tend to *arrest* a person in mid-excitement, or immediately following the peak of excitement.[54] (Italics mine)

Dr. Sacks goes on to state unequivocally,

> The vast majority of patients with incessant unremitting migraines are not the victims of ... physiological stimuli or sensitivities, but are caught in a malignant emotional 'bind' of one sort or another...[55]
>
> Thus a rage-migraine may be regarded as a complex but stereotyped reaction, in patients who experience this ... the patient is stuffed, impacted, and bloated with anger. The resolution of the attack may proceed by crisis (brief forceful vomiting, sudden passage of flatus and faeces, sneezing, etc.) or by lysis (diuresis, diaphoresis, epiphora, etc.). Thus the rage of such attacks is

> expressed in plethora, and discharged with sudden visceral ejaculation ... or a slow secretory catharsis...[56]

Finally, Dr. Sacks himself succinctly sums us that "migraine shows itself both eloquent and effective in providing an oblique expression of feelings which are denied direct or adequate expression in other ways."[57]

Rose and Gavel's second group of trigger factors are exhaustion, exercise, and sex. Migraines can lead to extreme prostration and exhaustion, but they can also be triggered by over-fatigue. Likewise, more than normal physical activity can trigger a migraine in some people. Sex also may trigger a migraine.[58] This may occur with or directly after orgasm in both men and women. It is also not uncommon for both men and women to experience sexual arousal before or during a migrainous attack for no "explainable" reason.

> A recent study in Florence, Italy has confirmed what many sufferers know but seldom talk about -- even to their doctors. And that is that a significant proportion of migraine sufferers experience intense sexual arousal as one of the body's chemical reactions during an attack. It may occur at the beginning of the process but happens more often towards the end, especially if the attack has lasted for days.[59]

Paradoxically, both exercise and sex in other individuals or at other times may actually alleviate incipient migraines.

Irregular meals mans skipping meals for longer than usual periods. Fasting here means skipping of meals for an even longer period of time. Both may provoke migraines in certain individuals who have a tendency to hypoglycemia. Prof. Rudolfo Low believes that all migraineurs are basically hypoglycemic.[60] While this may be a bit of an over-simplification, certainly hypoglycemia does play a part in the migraine scenario.

Rose and Gavel place alcohol with fasting and irregular meals as a triggering factor. I would place it under certain triggering foods. Nonetheless, alcohol use may both trigger and aggravate a migraine in certain persons. Some migraine sufferers may attempt to deaden their pain by getting drunk the way Ulysses S. Grant did. However, alcohol is no cure or palliative and only makes the situation worse.

Smoking nicotine can also trigger a migraine in some people, and there are many foods which act as migraine stimuli. But, interestingly, not all foods will trigger migraines in all people. Various individual's migraines are triggered by only certain foods. Dr. Edda Harrington, in surveying a group of 500 migraineurs, found that the following percentages of that group avoided the following foods as possible migraine precipitants:[61]

Chocolate	74%
Cheese & dairy	47%
Fruit, esp. citrus	30%
Alcohol, esp. red wine	25%
Fried, fatty foods	18%
Vegetables (variety unspecified)	18%
Tea and/or coffee	15%
Meat, exp. pork	14%
Seafood, meaning shellfish	10%

Some Western researchers and clinicians have rejected such lists of foods as causative or triggering factors since not even the same food will trigger a migraine headache every time in a given individual. Certainly, foods can be and often are a complicating factor in migraines. Rose and Gavel estimate, however, that less than 10% of migraines are due to food.[62] Rose and Gavel give the following example of a typical migraineur's relationship with an offending food: "One migraine subject always had an attack of headache some hours after eating pork, but only when tired or under emotional stress, and could eat pork with impunity if in 'good condition'..."[63] This suggests that food is a co-factor in triggering migraines bit is not the whole story. Happily, as we shall see further on, Chinese medicine can explain why any given patient's migraine may be triggered by any particular food.

It is well known that changes in sleep/wake cycle can precipitate migraines. If a person's migraine is triggered by fatigue, staying up too late may set the headache off. However, more often over-sleeping is responsible. Western medicine finds this paradoxical. Chinese medicine explains this easily.

We have already seen how many women's migraines are related to either the onset or the cessation, whether monthly or at menopause, of their periods and we will examine the traditional Chinese explanations for this in some detail. Likewise, oral contraceptives may precipitate or worsen the tendency to migraines in many women. Dr. James W. Lance says, "Birth control pills tend to increase the severity and the occurrence of migraines."[64] Again, Chinese medicine has a clear explanation of this. In such women, the first, obvious step is to discontinue the Pill.

Glare, weather changes, and external cold are all known to trigger migraines in certain individuals. Glare can be natural light reflected off roads and water, simply very bright sunlight, or exposure to strong artificial light. The flickering light of poor flourescents seems to be especially aggravating to migraine sufferers. Weather changes which can precipitate migraines may be either low or high pressure fronts. Low pressure fronts are associated with damp, humid weather. High pressure fronts may be associated with hot, dry winds. Either may precipitate migraines in certain individuals. Western medicine is perplexed by this seeming paradox, but Chinese medicine explains it easily.

Hot baths and exposure to cold, including eating very cold things, such as ice cream and frozen yogurt, can also trigger a migraine. Again, this seems paradoxical. However, once one knows something about the energetic mechanisms of how a migraine is produced, these seeming contradictions are relatively easily explained. It does not mean that exposure to cold or heat will always trigger an attack in each and every migraineur. In Chinese medicine, knowing that an individual person's attacks are triggered by either hot or cold helps to establish their Chinese diagnosis.

Rises in blood pressure or hypertension can trigger migraine attacks. So also can toothaches, sinusitis, and trigeminal neuralgia. Likewise, traumatic injury to the head may also initiate an attack or predispose a person to attacks who never had them before. As we will see below, simple tension headache may also trigger or turn into migraines.

And finally, head colds and hayfever or upper respiratory allergies may also precipitate a migraine headache. Based on all these triggering stimuli and their diversity, it is obvious that the migraine process is quite complex and multifaceted. It is no simple, discrete process but a complicated web of relationships. Depending upon the exact configuration of these relationships in a given individual at a certain age, time, or geographic place, various different factors may trigger their headache and also shape its symptoms and course. As Willis in the seventeenth century correctly perceived, migraines may be triggered by: "An evil or weak constitution of the parts ...sometimes innate and hereditary ... an irritation of some distant member or viscera ... changes of season, atmospheric states, the great aspects of the sun and moon, violent passions, and errors in diet."[65]

EPILEPSY AND MIGRAINES

For hundreds, if not thousands of years, clinicians have noticed the similarities between migraines and epilepsy. Both are species of attacks which are preceded by auras and seem to come out of nowhere. The auras of both may be "characterized by hallucinations of smell, feelings of *deja vu*, and sometimes forced reminiscence and forced affect."[66] Likewise it is possible in both instances to have numbness and tingling, convulsions and tremors, and loss of consciousness. Only a little more than a hundred years ago, both were referred to as forms of apoplexy.

However, because of the stigma attached historically to epilepsy, most modern writers have steered clear of this touchy subject. Be that as it may, I think there is a relationship between epilepsy and migraines as Chinese medicine will explain below. Sacks, in discussing the fact that some migraines are accompanied by muscular spasm and tremor, asks,

> How should we characterize such an attack? As atypical migraines with migrainous convulsions, as atypical epilepsies with migrainoid features, or as attacks of epilepsy superimposed on migraines?[67]

Hughlings Jackson, attempting to desensitize this topic, adds,

> While scientifically migraine is, I think, to be classified with epilepsies ... it would be absurd to classify it along with ordinary cases of epilepsy as to class whales with other mammals for the purposes of practical life. A whale is in law a fish; in zoology it is a mammal.[68]

Although the disease mechanisms of epilepsy and migraines are related, still there are differences in their course and it is not appropriate in either clinical practice or everyday life to equate as identical the two.

THE WORST CASE SCENARIO OF MIGRAINE

Migraine sufferers experience such terrible pain, they often feel as if their heads were going to split or explode or their eyes pop out. Therefore, it is not uncommon for migraineurs to worry about long-term or serious damage from their attacks. Instances of permanent damage from migraine are "exceedingly rare". However, there are instances of hemianopia (blindness in one eye), hemiplegia (paralysis of one side), hemisensory deficits (one-sided loss of various senses), and subarachnoid (under the skull) and cerebral (inside the brain) bleeding. I mention this not to scare migraine sufferers but because those rare occurrences do also establish a connection between the disease mechanism of migraines with stroke or what is now more commonly referred to as CVA (cerebral vascular accident). We will look at this connection further on when we come to explain according to Chinese medical theory each and every one of the Western medical facts presented in this section.

DIFFERENTIATION OF MIGRAINE FROM OTHER TYPES OF HEADACHE

Tension Headaches

It is necessary, at least in Western medicine, to differentiate migraines from other types of headaches, especially tension headaches, sinus headaches, and brain tumor headaches. Tension headaches are due to muscular tightening of the muscles of the upper back, neck, and scalp. Tension headaches tend to be insidious in their onset, directly related to stress and tension in one's life, and are characterized by a tight feeling as opposed to the piercing or pounding pain often associated with migraines. In some cases, tension headaches themselves may precipitate migraine attacks.

> Sometimes tension headache *and* migraine are experienced. In some cases the tension headache triggers the migraine ... On other occasions, a tension headache may develop out of a migraine attack, as the sufferer contracts the muscles of the neck and shoulders in an attempt to keep pain-inducing movements of the head to a minimum. This condition is a called a *mixed headache* in medical language...[69]

Like migraines, tension headaches tend to be more common in women than men.[70]

Sinus Headaches

Some headaches are due to inflammation and impaction of the sinus cavities which are like caves within the bones of the face. These spaces within the bones are connected to the nose and respiratory passages and infections and inflammations may establish themselves in these *cul de sacs*. Patients may experience a deep, pressury pain in the areas of these sinuses with or without any changes in nasal discharge. If the inflammation is occluded or hidden within, there does not have to be any purulent nasal mucous or traces of blood in the mucous. Sinuses are located over the eyes, above the bridge of the nose, and within the cheek bones. Therefore, one may experience the pressure of sinus headache in any or all of these areas.

Brain Tumor Headaches

If a person has hitherto not experienced migraine and then suddenly has a severe attack, it is not uncommon for that person to fear that they have a brain tumor. Their pain is so intense and unlike anything they have felt before, they are sure that something equally serious is going on within them. Because they hurt so much that they may want to die, they also fear that they may die. Therefore, it is also useful to know what the symptoms of brain tumor are in order to be able to rest easy that, no matter how bad the migrainous pain may be, one does not have a life-threatening tumor growing inside their head.

Typically, headaches associated with brain tumors have a history of short duration or recent onset but increasing severity. The headache is worse with coughing, sneezing, or bending over. The headache may wake the person from sleep and tends to be worse in the morning upon arising. It may be accompanied by or related to nausea and vomiting, especially in the AM. Often, there is associated drowsiness, yawning, and hiccup. If there are other neurological signs and symptoms, further investigation is mandatory.[71]

THE WESTERN MEDICAL TREATMENT OF MIGRAINES

Dr. James W. Lance, MD, states that, "There is no form of treatment of migraine that may be considered a cure, just as there is no cure for asthma or many other illnesses."[72] Generally, Western medicine attempts to treat migraines with various synthetic drugs. Of these, ergotamine, methysergide, clonidine, and propanolol are the four most commonly prescribed.

Ergotamine is prescribed to alleviate the pain of a migraine in progress. According to Dr. Sacks, "If ergotamine is going to work *at all*, it must be given very promptly, before the headache is established..."[73] However, ergotamine, sold under a number of propietary brand names including Ergomar, Ergostat, Bellergal, Cafergot, and Wigraine, is an extremely dangerous drug and unfortunately it is easy for its users to over-dose on it. If a little doesn't work, migraine sufferers are likely to take twice as much more and then more again, desperately seeking relief from the pounding and throbbing in their heads. This drug is so dangerous that it can cause gangrene of the intestines and of the hands and feet. Unfortunately, 50% of migrainous ergotamine users experience adverse reactions from this drug[74], including nausea, vomiting, diarrhea, cold hands and feet, chest and muscle pain, headache, dizziness, and confusion.[75]

> The problem with ergotamine is that, as work at specialist migraine clinics over the past few years has revealed, an effective dose is only a little less than a dose that produces side-effects, the most common of which are nausea, vomiting, headache, diarrhea, and a general feeling of being unwell.[76]

Methysergide is prescribed to prevent the occurrence of migrainous attacks or to reduce their frequency and severity. It is sold under the name Sansert in the United States. It is a serotonin-blocking drug, serotonin being a neurochemical found in the brain. Methysergide likewise has many side-effects, such as weight gain and fluid retention, skin rashes, temporary scalp hair loss, heartburn, nausea, vomiting, diarrhea, drowsiness, dizziness, urinary disturbance, and even nightmares, hallucinations, and acute mental disturbance.[77]

> At present we do not know precisely how it works. But we do know for certain that it is as dangerous as it is effective, with very serious and far-reaching side-effects if not used with extreme care by doctors and patients.[78]

Propanolol is an anti-hypertensive drug which is sold in the United States under the names Inderol and Inderide. It is one of the so-called Beta-blocking medicinals developed in the last decade or so. Besides being used to prevent migraine headaches, it is used in the treatment of angina pectoris, high blood pressure, and heart arrhythmias. It should not be taken by anyone with hayfever or a tendency to asthma. Its so-called natural unavoidable side-effects are lethargy, fatigue, cold hands and feet, and dizziness when one stands up. Its mild, unexpected adverse reactions include skin rashes, temporary balding, reduced appetite, nausea, vomiting, diarrhea, insomnia, vivid dreaming, and drug-induced fever. Its serious adverse reactions are disorientation, confusion, hallucinations, amnesia, depression, and increased risk of asthma. If a moderate overdose of propanolol is taken, it will cause general weakness, a slow pulse, and dizziness on arising (orthostatic hypotension). A large overdose will cause fainting, cold, sweaty skin, a weak, slow pulse, and even convulsions.[79] Obviously, this drug is also quite dangerous and somewhat unpredictable.

Clonidine, sold as Catapres, Combipres, and Dixarit, is also a fairly recent anti-hypertensive drug. It has many of the same side-effects as methysergide and propanolol. However, its natural, expected side-effects also include dry mouth and nose and constipation. As for its unexpected side-effects, it can cause dry, burning eyes, breast distention, water retention, and even temporary sexual impotence.[80] Clonidine is, like propanolol, used to prevent the occurrence and diminish the frequency and severity of migraines. All four of these drugs are available only by prescription and at least three cannot be stopped suddenly but must be withdrawn on a careful schedule. Otherwise, there may be withdrawal or rebound reactions.

Dr. Sacks suggests that the trend in U.S. migraine specialty clinics is towards "over-medication, over-investigation, and over-interference generally, coupled with an insufficient sense of the patient as an adult, and a responsible adult and agent in regard to his own welfare."[81] It is Dr. Sacks' opinion that Western medicine will never find a single medicine that will cure migraines categorically and he holds this opinion for two reasons:

> 1) There does not seem to be any single, invariable mechanism for the production of migraines. A migraine is a highly distinctive physiological event, and yet it is one that may be reached in a variety of ways...

2) The second reason is that though a migraine is a physiological event, it is not *just* a physiological event, but one that tends to be strongly related to, and determined by, the affected *individual* -- his character, his 'needs', his circumstances, and his mode of life. Thus it is insufficient to look for purely physiological remedies, when what one may have to remedy, if it can be remedied, is a whole way of life, a whole life.[82]

This echoes Gowers' nineteenth century view that, "Measures that do good in one case will fail in another, apparently quite similar."[83] Although this is a holistic vision of migraine which identifies the condition with the individual, still it leads Dr. Sacks and Western medicine to offer relatively little in terms of safe and effective, long-term, preventive treatment. Rather, he counsels a very conservative approach to the management of individual attacks:

Coffee or strong tea, rest, silence, and darkness
A simple analgesic, such as aspirin 'or something comparable'
An anti-emetic if there is nausea
And mild sedatives, such as phenobarbitol, librium, or valium to relieve the 'pathological excitements' -- the pounding head, the irritability, the restlessness, the anxiety...[84]

Caffeine, aspirin, phenobarbitol, librium, and valium may be quantitatively safer than ergotamine, methysergide, propanolol, and clonidine; however, each of these drugs also have their side-effects and, with the exception of aspirin, I would hesitate to call any of them benign medications. Although they might be safely employed without side-effects if Western medicine had a truly distinctive differential diagnosis of individual patient's migraines, since Western medicine does not, its use of such powerful drugs all too often does cause side-effects and drug reactions. In Appendix II, we will discuss a wiser use of these drugs based on Chinese diagnostic and pharmaceutical theory.

Some Western doctors do put their migraine sufferers on various diets. Usually this is based on some theory of allergy or histamine avoidance. Unfortunately, again because Western medicine does not understand the energetic mechanisms of migraine headaches, its dietary prohibitions tend to be too general and, therefore, too restrictive. It cannot say exactly who should avoid what foods and when for a good enough reason. Therefore, its patients often have difficulty complying with an overly exclusive regime which limits their diet too strictly.

In the last two decades, some Western researchers and clinicians have been using biofeedback as a way to prevent and lessen migraine attacks in many patients. This is a step in the right direction. However, biofeedback alone does not work for everyone. It tends to be used in clinics where physicians recognize the drawbacks of Western drug therapy as currently prescribed. But, using biofeedback alone falls into the same dichotomy of separating body and mind as using drug therapy alone. Saying that migraines are psychosomatic and then only addressing the psyche is just as extreme and one-sided as only treating the soma or body. As we will see further on, Chinese medicine treats the psyche and soma as an indivisible unit, and in such a truly holistic medicine, biofeedback and similar relaxation techniques play an important role. As Dr. Sacks rightly says,

> That one may learn to intervene, in this way, and modify one's own erring or aberrant responses, is now well-established ... The *idea* of biofeedback is genuine self-help, enabling the patient to achieve active mastery and control of himself...[85]

Modern Western medicine also, in a few instances, recommends the surgical removal of the affected superficial arteries in cases of intractable migraine. This is based on the idea that if something cannot be fixed any other way and that something is not absolutely necessary to the continuance of life, one can remove that something and, therefore, remove the problem altogether. Although I also would not disagree that in a scant percentage of intractable cases, surgical excision is also warranted even by Chinese medical theory, surgery most definitely does not remove the problem. Migraine is a complex internal process and simply removing the site of its symptomatic expression does not and cannot abort that process itself. The process will continue and must find another area or site to express itself in some other, although related sign or symptom.

Dr. Sacks, whom I obviously feel is the most perceptive contemporary Western medical author on migraines, sums up for me the limitations of modern Western medicine in dealing with this disease.

> The present century has been characterized both by advances and retrogressions in its approach to migraine. The advances reflect sophistication of technique and quantitation, and the retrogressions represent the splitting and fracturing of the subject which appears inseparable from the specialization of knowledge. By historical irony, a real gain of knowledge and technical skill has been coupled with a real loss in general understanding.[86]

In contradistinction, the Western clinical observers of the eighteenth century, such as Tissot, Whytt, Cheyne, Cullen, and Sydenham, "made no arbitrary distinctions between the physical and emotional aspects: all had to be considered together, as integral parts of 'nervous disorders'."[87]

Dr. Sacks, writing in 1985, is very clear about what medicine should be and what Western medicine is not:

> There is a tendency, increasingly, to reduce Medicine to medicines; to reduce, and to regard as irrelevant or 'old-fashioned' any personal attention to the patient, and to treat, in a purely mechanical way, (a patient's) physiological disorder. This is the *mood* of our harried, hurried, drug-hungry, Modern Medicine. But it is a mood that is hostile to the proper treatment of migraine -- or, as one should say, to the treatment of migraine *patients*. For it is not the migraine, but the *patient*, who needs treatment. The proper treatment of

> migraine, then, although it will make fullest use of whatever new discoveries and new techniques become available, must always turn and return to the affected *individual*, and finds its heart in an 'old-fashioned', *personal* attention.[88]
>
> It is neither a technique nor a 'treatment' which the physician finally gives, though his giving must include techniques and treatments. What must finally be given is understanding -- and courage: an *attitude* that is life-affirming in the face of disease. The patient requires *strength*, so he can stand up alone, and then, and only then, can he dispense with the physician, because in self-understanding, self-help, he can now be physician to himself. Thus Medicine, which may first need to come from others, from the outside, must activate an inner power, a Healing Will, in the patient, and when this occurs (and one can only hope it occurs!) one's migraines, one's illness, loose their baleful sting.[89]

It is my experience that traditional Chinese medicine has kept alive the general but nonetheless clinically precise enough understanding of the process of migraines which Western medicine has lost. In addition, Chinese medicine always treats the individual, both body and mind, as a unity, an inseparable and organic whole. Further, Chinese medicine treats the individual and not some abstract concept of a disease entity. But even more importantly, Chinese medical theory vis a vis the migraine process can bring great self-understanding to migraine sufferers. I agree with Dr. Sacks that it is precisely such self-understanding, which leads to self-help and self-responsibility, that is a medical theory's most important gift it can bestow on its patients.

Traditional Chinese medicine can explain all the idiosyncracies and vagaries of migraine in a way which no other medicine of which I am aware can. Its explanations empower its patients and lead eventually to transcendence of dependence upon its technical therapies. And, its theories are so general and universally descriptive that even a two thousand plus year old, ‘old-fashioned’ medicine can encompass and bring wisdom and discrimination to the use of Western medicine’s most modern drugs and procedures.

CHINESE MEDICAL THEORIES GERMANE TO UNDERSTANDING MIGRAINE

In Chinese medicine there is a basic axiom: *Tong Ze Bu Tong; Bu Tong Ze Tong* if there is free flow, there is no pain; if there is pain, there is no free flow. This statement covers every type of pain anywhere in the body due to any cause. When Qi (energy) and Blood flow easily and unobstructedly through the body, there is no pain. If there is pain, this is the subjective sensation of the blockage of Qi and Blood flow. Although, as we will see below, there are many ways the flow of Qi and Blood may become obstructed or impatent, there is no other cause of pain beyond impatency of the Qi and Blood.

THE CIRCULATION OF QI & BLOOD

According to Chinese medical theory, Qi and Blood circulate through the body over discrete Channels and through distinct Vessels. These Channels and Vessels are called collectively the *Jing Mai*. They form a continuous, closed loop similar but not identical to the Western vasculature. This net or web of pathways is made up of large Channels (*Jing*) which branch into smaller Collaterals, called *Luo Mai*, and these *Luo* branch into even smaller Collaterals called *Sun Luo*. *Sun Luo* are analogous to the capillary beds in Western medicine.

There are twelve main or so-called Regular Channels (*Shi Er Zheng Jing*) which traverse the body and distribute Qi and Blood to and from the Organs and Bowels in the Interior and the extremities at the Exterior. Each of these Twelve Regular Channels (which are themselves symmetrically bilateral) connects with one of the twelve basic Organs of Chinese medicine. Therefore, these Channels are often referred to by the name of the Organ or Bowel with which they connect. For instance, we may speak of the Liver Channel or Meridian, the Heart Channel, the Stomach Channel, etc. However, because each one of these Channels begins or ends on either the hands or feet and because these Channels are also paired, one Hand Channel being contiguous with one Foot Channel, in Chinese medicine we also often speak if the Six Channels (*Liu Jing*).

When we divide up the Twelve Regular Channels into six pairs, we get:

Tai Yang (Maximum Yang) = Small Intestine & Bladder
Shao Yang (Lesser Yang) = Gallbladder & Triple Heater
Yang Ming (Bright Yang) = Stomach & Large Intestine
Tai Yin (Maximum Yin) = Lung & Spleen
Jue Yin (Exhausted Yin) = Liver & Pericardium
Shao Yin (Lesser Yin) = Heart & Kidney

Four of these six pairs are classically used to describe pain in the major regions of the head. Pain at the base of the skull in the back or occipital region is due to obstruction or impatency of the flow of Qi and Blood in the *Tai Yang*. Pain in the sides of the head or temporal regions is due to a problem with the circulation of the *Shao Yang*. Pain in the forehead or frontal region is related to the

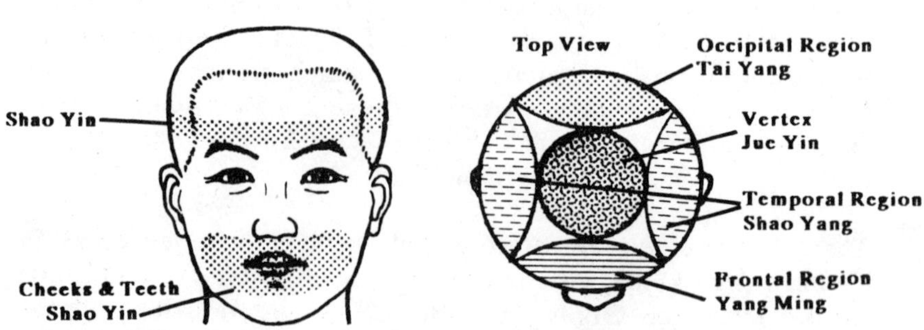

Figure 1.
Energetic Regions of the Head

Yang Ming. And pain at the crown of the head or vertex is ascribed to the *Jue Yin*. In addition, although most traditional Chinese discussions of head pain do not mention the remaining two of the six pairs, we can say that pain like a band all around the head pertains to the *Tai Yin*, and that pain in the cheeks and teeth pertains to the *Shao Yin*. Fig. 1 shows the six areas of the head described above. Figs. 2-13 (p. 40-42) show the pathways of the Twelve Regular Channels.

REASONS FOR IMPATENCY OF THE QI & BLOOD

There are a number of reasons why the circulation of Qi and Blood may become impatent or not free flowing in the regions of the head. However, these may be divided into three broad categories:

Blockage
Excess
Deficiency

BLOCKAGE

Blockage means that something is occupying the space of the Channels and, therefore, the Qi and Blood which normally flow through that space cannot. They back up behind this obstruction and the pressure this causes is experienced as pain. The factors which may cause blockage to the free and unobstructed flow of Qi and Blood through the Channels and Vessels of the head are:

1) Externally invading pathogens
2) Internally produced pathological substances
3) Traumatic injury

Headache Due To External Pathogens

Chinese medicine believes that pathogens from the outside environment can invade the body and lodge in the Channels and Collaterals. Chinese medicine speaks of these pathogens as Evil Qi (*Xie Qi*) or Evil Winds (*Feng Xie*). Headache can arise if Evil Wind Cold, Wind Heat, or Wind Dampness invade the Channels

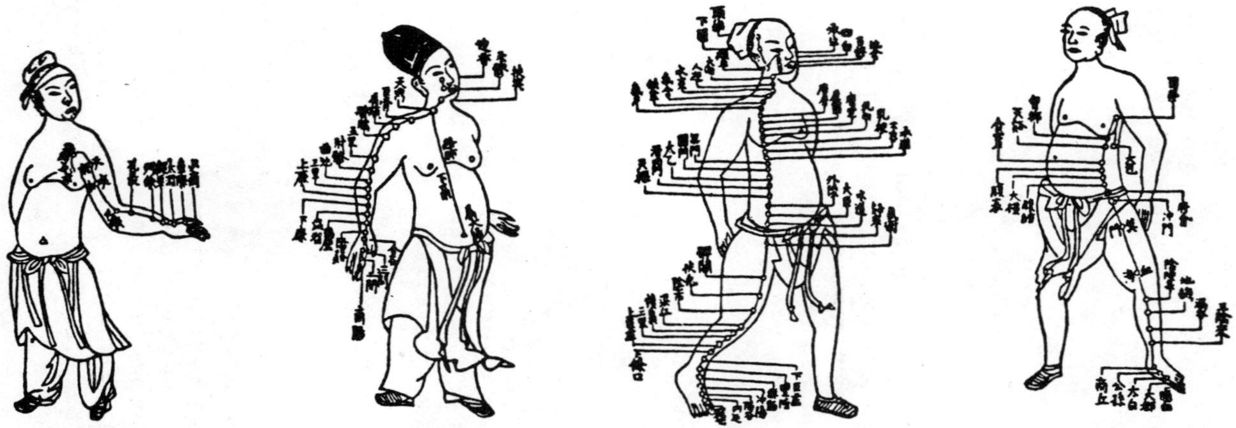

手太阴肺經 Lung Meridian

手阳明大腸經 Large Intestine Meridian

足阳明胃經 Stomach Meridian

足太阴脾經 Spleen Meridian

Figure 2-5.

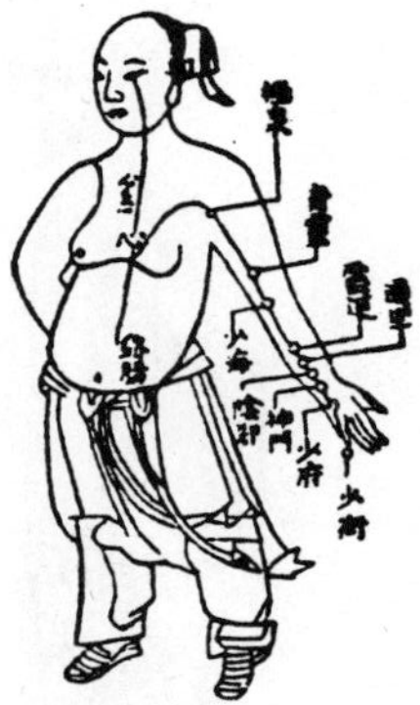

Heart Meridian

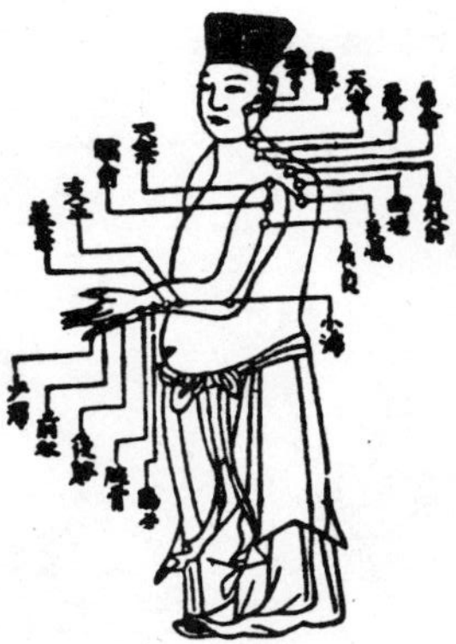

Small Intestine Meridian

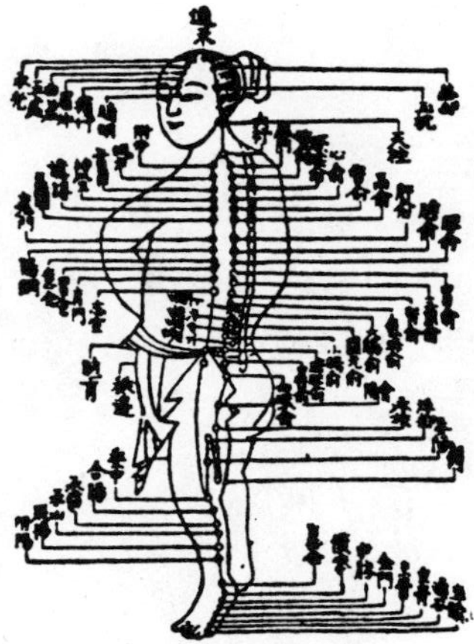

Bladder Meridian

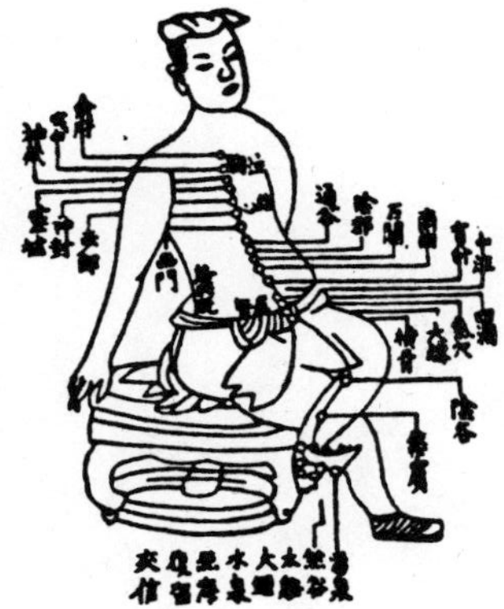

Kidney Meridian

Figure 6-9.

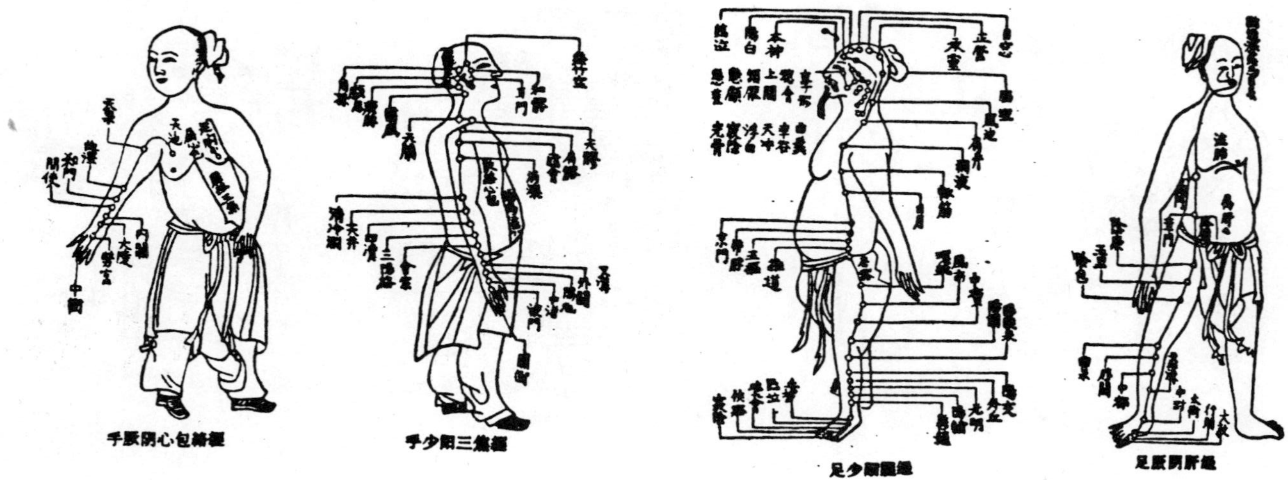

Pericardium Meridian Triple Heater Meridian Gall Bladder Meridian Liver Meridian

Figure 10-13.

and Collaterals of the head. Wind, in this context, means some unseeable pathogen. Cold, Heat, and Dampness describe the body's manifestation of dis-ease in the same language that one might describe a storm moving through the external environment. It is not that cold has caused the dis-ease, but rather that the dis-ease manifests similar to cold outside. When this happens, the Wind Evils occupy the space within which the Qi and Blood must flow and now cannot.

Based on theory too complicated to go into here, a Wind Cold invasion can effect the whole head, just the back of the head or occiput, or just the left side of the head. A Wind Heat invasion can effect the sides of the head bilaterally or just the right side alone. And a Wind Damp invasion typically feels like a tight band wrapped around the head or the whole head may feel very heavy. Such Wind Evil invasions are similar to the Western concepts of catching a cold, a chill, or a draft. They can correspond to colds and flues, hayfever, and allergies, and a number of other acute, relatively transient complaints in Western medicine.

Headache Due To Internal Pathological Substances

Internally generated pathological substances which may lodge in and block the pathways of the head are:

1) Dampness
2) Phlegm
3) Stagnant Blood

Dampness is produced when either or all the Lungs, Spleen, and Kidneys fail to transform and transport Liquids properly. In this case, a pathological accumulation of Liquids becomes Dampness. If Dampness is drafted up into the head, it may obstruct and retard the flow of Qi and Blood. When this happens, one experiences a stuffy, full head or a band of tension around the head similar to Wind Dampness.

Phlegm is a further condensation of pathologic Dampness. If Dampness lingers or is stewed by Heat within the body, it may congeal or condense into Phlegm. This Phlegm can then block the flow of Qi and Blood through the *Jing Luo* giving rise to dull pain, dizziness, and even loss of consciousness. Phlegm and Dampness or Fluids often exist together, in which case they are called in Chinese medicine *Tan Yin* .

Stagnant Blood is Blood which no longer flows through its Vessels. If anything causes retardation in the flow of Qi and Blood for a long time, eventually the Blood will become Stagnant. This happens in the *Sun Luo* or small capillary-like Collaterals. This Stagnant Blood then further impedes the circulation of Qi and Blood and gives rise to pricking, sharp, stabbing or piercing pain.

Headache Due To Traumatic Injury

In Chinese medicine, it is believed that traumatic injury, whether a blow or a cut, causes a rupture in the Channels and Collaterals. The Qi and Blood flow out of their pathways and mull or puddle. Because the Qi and Blood are not canalized or channeled, they accumulate in the area of the injury and also cause obstruction to the flow of Body Fluids in the area. This causes swelling, inflammation, and pain. If an injury is not resolved completely, it may leave behind a residue of Stagnant Blood in the *Sun Luo* or capillaries. Such a residue may cause recurrent headache, especially if complicated by other factors.

EXCESS

In many cases, the body's metabolism produces too much of something and when there is too much, it all cannot fit within the Channels and Collaterals and be distributed without pressure and, therefore, pain. In general, what is Excess is Yang. Yang is a general concept for all that is airy, light, moving, functional, and warm. Yang is the energy of Heaven, as opposed to Yin, the energy of Earth. Therefore, all Yang energies tend to float or move upward. Yang is life which is evaporated or transformed from Yin. Yang is function and Yin is the substance which both roots and is the fuel for the Yang. Within the human body, Yang essentially is Qi. All Yang Excesses are an Excess of Qi. However, since Qi usually connotes life and health, when Qi itself causes disease, it is usually given another name. We can speak then of Congested Qi,

Heat, Ascendant Yang, or Internal Wind.

Congested Qi

Although Qi is life and is good, if it becomes congested or blocked, it may accumulate pathologically. When it does, eventually it will vent itself most typically upwards because it is Yang. The most common cause of Qi Congestion is stress. Under stress, we tighten ourselves and this constricts the free and patent flow of Qi. In Chinese medicine, it is the Liver which is responsible for maintaining the free and easy flow of Qi and it is the Liver where the Qi collects due to stress and emotional blockage.

In particular, anger and frustration congest the Qi and make it flow upward towards the head. Since the Liver is a Yin Organ and Qi is a Yang energy, accumulated, congested Qi is vented in to the paired Yang Bowel associated with the Liver, the Gallbladder. This Qi then flows upwards towards the head along the path of the Gallbladder Channel or *Shao Yang*.

Besides stress, anger, and emotional upset, the Qi can also be blocked and accumulate due to any of the other, so-called Six Stagnations. These are Qi, Blood, Food, Dampness, Phlegm, and Heat. If any of these other five accumulate, since they are all relatively more dense than the Qi, they tend to impede the flow of the Qi and cause Qi Stagnation as well. Conversely, since it is the Qi which transports and transforms Blood, Food, Dampness, Phlegm, and disperses Heat, if Qi flow becomes sluggish and congested, it often causes accumulation of one or more of these as well.

Essentially, the process of life is the transformation of substance or matter into energy and the transformation of this energy into consciousness. This is described in Chinese medicine as the interrelationship between *Jing* Essence (ultimate substance), Qi (energy or function), and *Shen* (Spirit or consciousness). Within the physical body, this transformation entails the ascension of the Qi to the upper body as it becomes *Shen*. Therefore, Qi naturally and should ascend to the Heavens (in the body, the head). however, if too much Qi, as opposed to transformed *Shen*, ascends to and accumulates in the head, it causes pain.

Heat

Qi has five functions in the human body: it transports or propels; it transforms; it warms; it defends; and it holds or restrains. Therefore, Qi is inherently Warm. If too much Qi accumulates in an area or Organ of the body, it may transform into an accumulation of Heat. Professional practitioners categorize a certain amount of Qi in one place as Heat, but it is essential to remember that this is merely a conceptual categorization and Heat is nothing other than Qi.

Typically, Heat tends to accumulate in certain specific Organs or areas of the body. These are the Liver, Stomach, Heart/Pericardium, Lungs, and Gallbladder. Likewise, Heat tends to move upwards. Even if Heat begins in the Liver or Stomach, it frequently tends to travel to and express itself in the head. Although it may also express itself as inflammation and ulceration, Heat, because it is none other than a lot of Qi, also often manifests as headache, i.e. too much Qi trying to travel through too little space. If the Heat is coming from the Liver, it may manifest as pain in the *Jue Yin* (vertex) or *Shao Yang* (Temporal regions). If Heat is arising from the Stomach, it may manifest as pain in the *Yang Ming* (frontal region). In addition, Heat in one Organ may give rise to or exacerbate Heat in another, closely related Organ. For instance, Liver and Stomach Heat often mutually aggravate each other.

Ascendant Yang

The Root of all Heat in the body, whether Righteous (normal) or Evil (pathologic) is the *Ming Men Zhi Huo*, the Life Gate Fire. This is the Yang Qi of the Kidneys, the Root Organs of the entire body. If Kidney Water, which is Yin, becomes weak or exhausted, Kidney Fire, which is Yang, will tend to float upwards collecting in and aggravating any tendency to Heat in the Liver, Gallbladder, Stomach, Heart/Pericardium, and/or Lungs. Eventually, this Heat often rises to and accumulates in the Head. This is Heat which arises due to Deficiency of Kidney Yin or a basic Excess of Yang and Deficiency of Yin. According to Chinese Yin Yang theory, if either Yin or Yang become Deficient, the other will tend to become Excess.

Therefore, Ascendant Yang is also another category describing too much Qi rising to the head. When a Chinese doctor speaks of Ascendant Yang, we most often are referring to Liver Yang. In Chinese medicine it is said, "The Liver tends to Excess." That is because the Liver easily becomes congested as described above due to stress or any of the other five Stagnations. This Qi may not transform into Heat per se, but may merely vent itself upwards. If part of this upward venting of Qi is due to insufficient Liver Blood and Kidney Yin holding or magnetizing this Qi in the lower half of the body, we call it Ascendant Yang (*Shang Yang*). However, whether we call it Congested Qi, Heat, or Ascendant Yang, it is ultimately nothing other than Qi.

Internal Wind

Likewise, if Qi is pent-up in the Liver and then it vents very suddenly or strongly upwards, this is referred to as Internal Stirring of Liver Wind (*Gang Feng Nei Dong*). Such Liver Wind tends to vent again upwards along the *Jue Yin* or *Shao Yang*. In addition, Internal Wind may be caused, in part, by Heat or may give rise to Heat just as in the outer environment wind can spread of fire or be generated by fire. Headaches associated with Internal Wind are rapid in onset, changeable in nature and location, and may be associated with tinnitus, dizziness, vertigo, convulsions, spasticity, and tingling, all of which in Chinese medicine are due to Qi running amok like a gust of strong wind.

DEFICIENCY

Blockage and Excess both cause pain due to an abnormal accumulation within the Channels and Collaterals which is easy to visualize and understand. Pain due to Deficiency is a little more difficult to understand. The Qi and Blood not only travel through the *Jing Mai* but, in a sense, also keep these open and 'inflated'. If the Qi or Blood become insufficient to maintain the openings of the Channels and Vessels, these collapse or close. When they collapse, this blocks or obstructs the flow of whatever Qi and Blood is trying to get through. This, in turn, causes light but insidious or continuous pain which is especially worse when the Qi and Blood are even further depleted and, therefore, even less capable of keeping the pathways open. Typically, this type of headache worsens towards evening after the day's activities have consumed Qi and Blood, when fatigued, or when hungry. Hunger is the body's feedback mechanism requesting more fuel to transform into more Qi and Blood. Also, women who tend towards Qi and Blood Deficiency will experience an aggravation of this after menstruation which is a discharge of Blood.

In clinical practice, the professional practitioner must distinguish between Qi Deficiency, Blood Deficiency, and *Jing* or Essence Deficiency headaches. In the case of Qi Deficiency, there is not enough Qi to pump the Blood up to the head. In the case of Blood Deficiency, there is not enough Blood to fill the Vessels and keep them open. Often these two Deficiencies occur together, since the Qi and Blood are mutually interdependent, the Qi moving and making the Blood, the Blood nourishing and stabilizing the Qi.

Jing Deficiency means Kidney Yin Deficiency. Kidney Yin is also called *Zhen Yin* or True Yin. It is the Root of all Yin or Pure Substance in the body. Blood is created, in part, out of *Jing* Essence. *Jing* also creates the Marrow or *Sui*. Marrow in Chinese medicine means the deepest, most condensed form of tissue. The Brain is called the Sea of Marrow (*Sui Hai*). If the Blood and *Jing* are insufficient, the Sea of Marrow may become empty and this also causes pain. This pain is likewise worse in the evening, when fatigued, after menstruation, after sex (especially in a man), or after any food or activity which might weaken the Kidneys in general and the *Jing* in particular.

ZANG FU PHYSIOLOGY

In order to understand why a given person at a given time may experience head pain due to either Blockage, Excess, or Deficiency and also in order to understand all the other accompanying signs and symptoms associated with migraine, it is necessary to understand the basic functions and inter-relationships between the

Chinese Twelve Organs. This is because traditional Chinese medicine is a thoroughly holistic system where every part and piece is dependent upon every other part and piece. In Chinese medicine, there are Six *Zang* or Organs and Six *Fu* or Bowels. Therefore, *Zang Fu* physiology means the functions of these Twelve Organs and Bowels.

THE SIX *ZANG*

Zang literally means a treasury or warehouse. The *Zang* Organs are the Heart, Pericardium, Lungs, Spleen, Liver, and Kidneys. These Organs are Yin in nature in that they create and store nutrients and vital Essence and are solid in form. These Chinese Organs are not the same as the Western organs of the same English name. Although they often refer to the same anatomical structure, the Chinese Organ is described as having different, although logically consistent functions.

In Chinese medicine, the Heart has two main functions: 1) It controls the Blood and the Blood Vessels (*Mai*). This refers to the Heart's pumping of the Blood and the Heart's role in the creation of the Blood. In relation to headache, the Heart Qi must be sufficient to pump up Blood to the head and the Heart must also manufacture enough Blood to nourish the head, and 2) it controls the Spirit. This refers to the Heart's housing the *Shen* Spirit or being the seat or center of consciousness. The Spirit is nourished by Heart Blood or Yin. When there is sufficient Heart Blood and Yin, the Spirit is calm. When there is not, the Spirit is anxious, restless, and agitated. In contemporary Chinese medicine, the Pericardium is often not considered a separate *Zang* but rather is seen as an extension of the Heart. This is a complex issue since the Pericardium is also closely related to Liver and also Kidney function. When the Pericardium is subsumed under the Heart, one then speaks of Five *Zang* and Six *Fu*.

The Chinese Liver's functions are fourfold: 1) The Liver stores the Blood. It regulates the volume of Blood in circulation at any given time. 2) Closely related to the Liver's storage of Blood, it also maintains the patent and free flow of Qi. This means that the Liver maintains a) the smooth and even flow of the emotions, b) the smooth and even flow of peristalsis, and c) the smooth and even flow of the Blood and Liquids propelled by the Qi through the passageways of the Triple Heater. 3) The Liver stores the *Hun* or Psyche. The Psyche is the mental activity of the individual or ego. When Liver Qi is patent and Liver Blood is full, the Psyche is calm within the Liver. When the Psyche is not calm, this manifests as disturbances in dreaming, hallucinations, and irritability. 4) The Liver controls the *Jin* Sinews. The *Jin* Sinews are an energetic layer of tissue in Chinese medicine which includes the tendons, ligaments, and much other connective tissue. In Chinese medicine, movement is dependent upon the contractibility and flexibility of the *Jin*. When Liver Blood is sufficient, the Sinews are nourished and they are supple and relaxed. When it is not, the Sinews become dry and there is stiffness, spasticity, tremor, and convulsions. In addition, the Liver 'opens' into the eyes. Vision is largely dependent upon Liver Blood nourishing the eyes' capacity to see. However, vision itself is a Yang function and Excess Liver Yang can also create visual disturbances, especially in the sense of seeing 'more' than what we normally see.

The spleen in Western medicine is much less important than the Spleen in Chinese medicine. In Chinese medicine, the Spleen is one of the most important of all Twelve Organs. 1) The Spleen controls the entire process of digestion. It is in charge of creating Qi, Blood, and Body Fluids out of the foods and liquids eaten and drunk. This process is summarized in Chinese medicine as sending the Pure up and the Turbid down. The Pure Qi is sent to the Lungs to become Qi and the Pure Liquids are sent to the Heart to become Blood. 2) The Spleen holds. Holding or astringing is one of the five basic functions of the Qi and the Spleen is the Root of the Qi derived from food and liquids. The Spleen Qi specifically holds the Organs up against to force of gravity and also holds the Blood within its pathways. 3) The Spleen stores the *Yi* or Intention. This means the ability to form a desire and the desire to implement it. *Yi* also includes the ability to remember and then to move from past memory into the future. 4) The Spleen controls the Flesh and limbs. Flesh is *Ji Rou* in Chinese. It includes the fat and muscle in the sense of the body's rounded, full shape. The Spleen's control of the Flesh means that if Spleen function is normal in providing nutrients from digestion, one is neither emaciated or obese. The

Spleen's control of the four limbs means that there is enough Qi and Blood to create movement and warmth.

The Lungs have three main functions in Chinese medicine. 1) They control the Qi. Just as the Heart's control of the Blood means that the Heart pumps the Blood to the entire rest of the body, the Lungs' control of the Qi means that the Lungs disperse the Qi to the rest of the body. 2) The Lungs maintain the downward flow of Fluids. This is based on the Lungs' dispersion of Qi. The Qi transports the Fluids downwards for eventual evacuation from the Bladder. 3) The Lungs store the *Po* or animal vitality. Vitality or a dynamic approach to life is based on abundant Qi or energy. If the Lungs function correctly vis a vis respiration, there is abundant Qi and, therefore, one can be active and dynamic or full of *Po* vitality.

The Kidneys are called the Prenatal Organ in Chinese medicine. They are believed to be the primordial Organ out of which all the others embryologically evolve. The Kidneys have five major functions in Chinese medicine. 1) They store *Jing* Essence and *Yuan* Source Qi. Jing Essence is the Root of all Pure Substance in the body. It is the Root of all Yin. *Yuan* Source Qi is the Root of all function, transportation, and transformation in the body. *Yuan Qi* is the Root of all Yang. It is closely related to the Fire of the Gate of Life or the so-called Moving Qi Between the Kidneys. As such, the Chinese Kidneys are the organic basis for life itself, and maturation and aging are both dependent upon Kidney function. The former is the expression of the flourishing of the Kidneys and the latter is the expression of their decline. 2) The Kidneys generate *Sui* Marrow. *Sui* Marrow is another level of tissue within Chinese medicine. It is produced and nourished by Kidney *Jing*. In regarding headaches, the Brain is the Sea of Marrow and, as mentioned above, Kidney Deficiency may lead to headache due to Emptiness of the Sea of Marrow. 3) The Kidneys control Water. This means the Kidneys transport Pure Fluids upwards for nourishing the tissues and Turbid Fluids downwards for elimination. In addition, Kidney Qi is responsible for holding Fluids within the body, such as nasal mucous, vaginal discharge, semen, Intestinal fluids, menstrual Blood, urine, and perspiration. 4) The Kidneys co-ordinate respiration as an extension of Kidney

Qi's grasping function. The Kidneys must grasp and hold the Qi sent down by the Lungs. 5) The Kidneys store the *Zhi* Will. The Will means determination and willpower, the ability to stick to something over a period of time and tribulation. In addition, the Kidneys "open" into the ears and hearing problems often relate to Kidney function.

THE SIX *FU*

Fu literally means a government agency responsible for some specific area of administration. In contemporary Chinese medicine, the *Fu* Bowels are not as important as the *Zang*. Of the Six *Fu*, only two are given much attention these days therapeutically. They are the Stomach and Gallbladder, and these two are certainly the most important in terms of headache. However, it is useful to know something about all Six *Fu* Bowels, each of which is paired with a *Zang* Organ.

The Small Intestine is the *Fu* Bowel paired with the Heart. In this case, the Heart is Yin and Interior and the Small Intestine is Yang and Exterior. The Small Intestine's Chinese medical function is to "receive and contain" the digestate and to differentiate the usable from the unusable, especially vis a vis Liquids.

The Gallbladder is the Yang Bowel paired with the Yin Liver. It is the reservoir of Bile. Together with the Liver, the Gallbladder helps promote the smooth flow of Qi and Blood. It is the Gallbladder's release of stored Bile into the Intestines which maintains the patency of peristalsis. The relationship between the Liver and Gallbladder is closer than some of the other Interior/Exterior, *Zang Fu* relationships.

The Stomach is the *Fu* paired with the Spleen. The Stomach and Spleen work so closely together in digestion that often the term Spleen/Stomach (*Pi Wei*) is used to denote digestion as a whole. In Chinese medicine, the Stomach is the reservoir of food and liquids. It receives these and then "rottens and ripens" the digestate so it can be distilled and separated by the Spleen. The Stomach Qi flows down and the Spleen Qi up. The Stomach dislikes Dryness and the Spleen dislikes Damp. Therefore,

Stomach/Spleen function is based on mutual co-ordination and complementation.

The Large Intestine is the Bowel paired with the Lungs. Similar to the other Bowels, the Large Intestine in general conveys and transforms. Whereas the Small Intestine primarily transforms liquids, the Large Intestine transforms food. The completely unusable portion or residue of the solid food is conveyed out of the body as feces by the Large Intestine.

The Bladder is paired with the Kidneys. It temporarily stores and then discharges urine similar to the bladder of Western medicine.

The Triple Heater (*San Jiao*) is paired with the Pericardium. However, the Triple Heater is not a separate anatomical organ as are the others. Rather, it represents the entire metabolism based on thé mutual co-ordination of all the other *Zang* and *Fu*. It is spoken of as a Bowel, since anatomically the Triple Heater is the upper, middle, and lower sections of the torso which contain the other *Zang Fu*. Therefore, the Triple Heater is "hollow" like the other Bowels. It is called Triple Heater because the three sections of the torso are called the Upper, Middle, and Lower Heaters. It is called Heater because, in Chinese medicine, all metabolic processes are recognized to be Warm transformations.

Although each *Zang* is paired with a specific *Fu* based on Interior/Exterior and Yin Yang relationships, various of the *Zang* and *Fu* have other close or mutually interdependent relationships. For instance, just as we have mentioned the close relationship between the Lungs and Kidneys, there is also a close relationship between the Heart and Kidneys. The Kidneys are the Root of Yang which arises to the Heart and is transformed into the *Shen Ming* or brilliance of consciousness. There is a close relationship between the Kidneys and the Liver based on the mutual relationship of *Jing* Essence and Blood. There is a close relationship between the Liver and Spleen vis a vis digestion, and another between the Liver and Lungs vis a vis ease of respiration and ascension and descension in the body as a whole. Likewise, the Liver and Stomach often mutually aggravate pathologic Heat within each other and the Liver and the Large Intestine Qi also tends to move together. And finally, the Heart and Spleen have a close relationship, the Spleen in terms of Qi production and the Heart in terms of Blood. Therefore, it is easy to see that, in Chinese medicine, all the Organs work synergistically and as a whole.

FIVE PHASE THEORY

In Chinese medicine, there is another theory or set of theories which help to describe the close interdependence of the Organs and their functions. This is called Five Phase Theory. Although this theory has been downplayed somewhat in contemporary Chinese medicine, it is very useful for understanding the various pathological relationships between the *Zang* and *Fu* in terms of all the signs and symptoms of migraine.

According to Five Phase Theory, each of the major Organs is associated with an Element or Phase. The Five Phases are Wood, Fire, Earth, Metal, and Water. These Five Phases both generate and also check and balance each other, both in the macorcosmic world outside and the microcosmic world internally. Therefore, likewise, the Organs both promote or generate each other and also check and inhibit each other according to definite, specific avenues of action.

Figure 14. Mother-Child Relationships

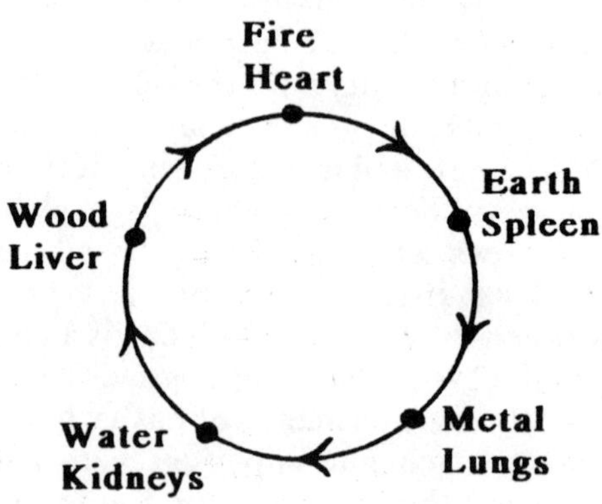

There are two major avenues of action or cycles of influence according to Five Phase Theory. The first is called the Creation or *Sheng* cycle. According to this cycle, the Liver, which is associated with the Wood Phase, is the mother of the Heart (Fire Phase) and the child of the Kidneys (Water Phase). That means the Liver receives its nourishment from the Kidneys and is responsible for giving sustenance to the Heart. Similarly, each of the five major Organs of Chinese medicine is the mother of one Organ and the child of another. These mother-child relationships are diagrammed in Figure 14.

The second cycle is called the Control or *Ke* cycle. It describes how the Phases and Organs check each other to maintain homeostasis. According to this cycle, Wood, i.e. the Liver, controls or checks Earth or the Spleen. Earth controls Water or the Kidneys. Water controls Fire or the Heart. Fire controls Metal or the Lungs. And Metal controls Wood or the Liver. These control or checking relationships are diagrammed below in Figure 15.

Figure 15. Control Cycle Checking Relationships

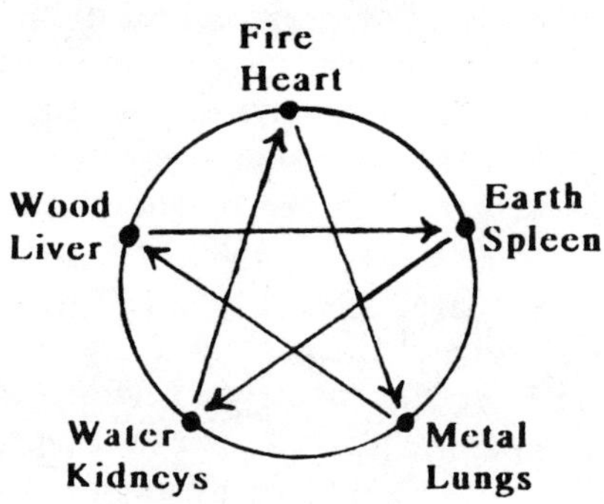

When we put both the *Sheng* and the *Ke* cycles together, we have a system of continuous generation with a built in mechanism to stop runaway proliferation. This self-correcting system of generation and control is diagrammed below in Figure 16.

Figure 16. Generation and Control Cycles operating simultaneously.

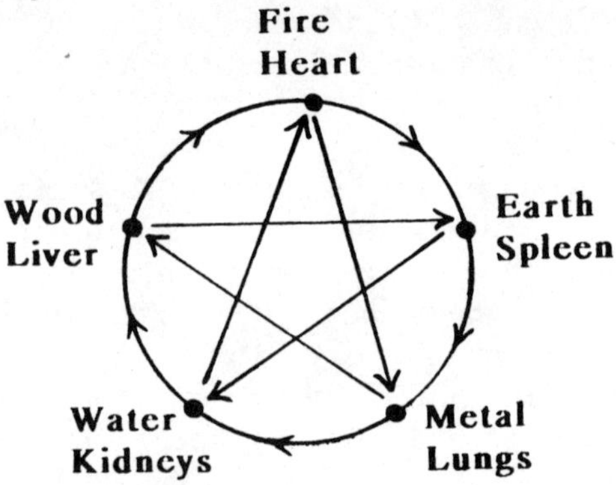

When this system operates correctly, it maintains the harmonious functioning of all the Organs and Bowels of the body. All are promoted but none are allowed to become too strong or out of balance. However, often, due to erroneous diet, lack of exercise, or emotional stress and over-fatigue, some Organs become too strong or Excess and others become too weak or Deficient. When this happens, disease will evolve also according to the avenues of action or influence described by the vectors of the *Sheng* and *Ke* cycles.

In Chinese medicine, one of the statements concerning the Liver is that, *Gan Zhu Sheng Fa*, the Liver governs development and expansion. This means that, when the Liver is functioning normally, it grows flourishingly like a tree in spring. However, it also implies that the Liver tends to proliferate. Another Chinese medical dictum reiterates this: *Mu Xi Taio Da*, Wood (the Liver) is inclined to flourish. Not only is the Liver inclined to Excess, but the Liver is the temperamental Organ in Chinese medicine. *Gan Wei Gang Zang* means the Liver is the "indomitable" Organ. It tends to be indomitable, Excess, and Hot.

When the Liver becomes Excess, it may cause symptoms of disease anywhere along the course of its Channel or along the course of its paired Bowel, the Gall Bladder's Channel. (See Figure 18.)However, it also sets in motion a number of changes in potentially all the other Organs depending upon such contributing factors as sex, diet, inherent constitutional tendencies, season of the year, phase of the moon, weather, stress, and rest. This explains Liver-related menstrual problems including dysmenorrhea, urinary problems, lower abdominal pain and distention, hypochondriac pain and distention, sciatica, flank pain, premenstrual nipple sensitivity, premenstrual irritability, lability, and depression, and premenstrual and one-sided headaches and headaches at the crown of the head.

If the Liver "invades" Earth along the path of the Control cycle, it may cause the Stomach to become Hot and Rebellious and/or the Spleen to become weak, Deficient, and also even Damp. This can manifest as Stomach upset, nausea, and vomiting on the one hand and diarrhea, painful bowel movements, intestinal upset, and constipation on the other. Since typically the Liver becomes more Excess just before the period, before its discharge of Blood from the Blood Chamber (the Uterus), this is also when women frequently experience signs and symptoms of the Liver's encroachment on the Stomach and Spleen.

Figure 17. Liver Wood invading the Stomach/Spleen

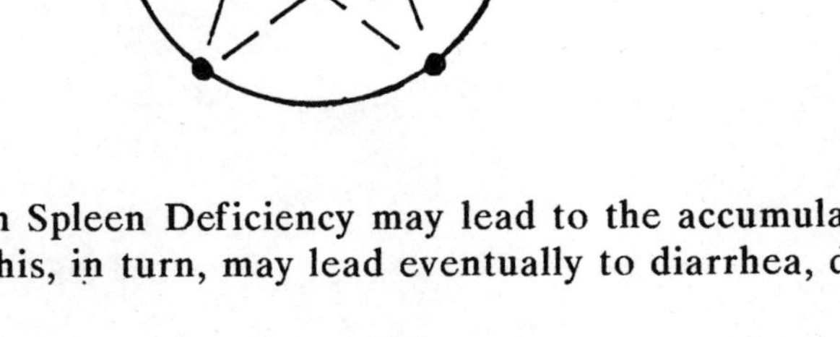

Long-term Spleen Deficiency may lead to the accumulation of Damp. This, in turn, may lead eventually to diarrhea, dysuria,

Figure 18.

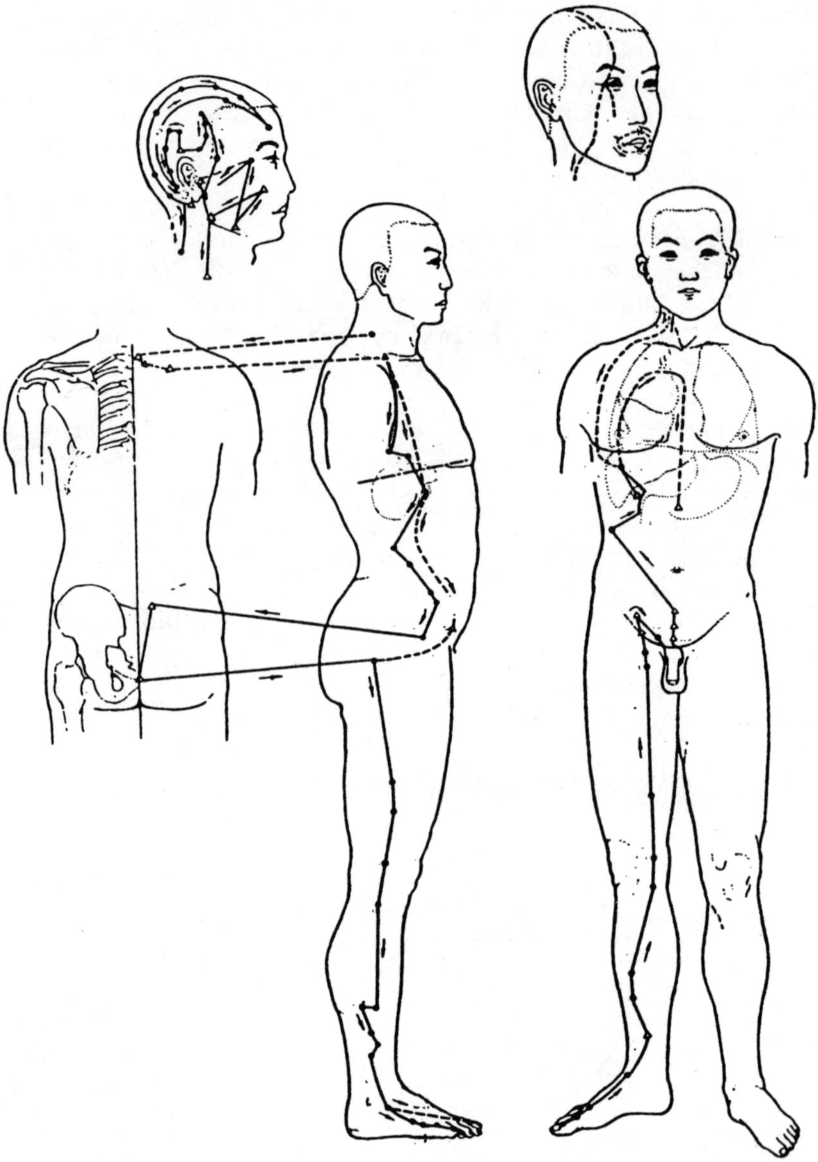

Course of the Gall Bladder Meridian **Course of the Liver Meridian**

polyuria, vomiting, leukorrhea, and a heavy sensation in the body in general and especially in the arms and legs. It may also cause headaches which feel like a band of tension surrounding the head. Any or all of these symptoms may become aggravated just before the period.

Long-term Spleen Deficiency may also lead to Blood Deficiency since it is the Spleen which initiates the creation of the Blood. This may lead to dysmenorrhea, hypomenorrhea, delayed menstruation, amenorrhea, and even infertility. It can also cause Blood Deficiency headache.

And further, since according to Chinese medicine it is the Spleen Qi which "lifts" or hold up all the other Organs, long-term Spleen Qi Deficiency may eventually result in prolapse of this so-called Central or Middle Qi. When this happens, the person experiences a bearing-down, dragging pain as if their insides were going to fall out and/or Qi Deficiency headache, fatigue, and dizziness. In terms of menstruation, this is most often experienced towards the end of menstruation when the woman has lost Blood and therefore also more Qi as well.

Since the Spleen is the mother of the Lungs, if the Spleen is weak, the Lungs will also become weak over time. Since the Lungs are supposed to control the Liver, this weakness allows the Liver to flourish or to become even more Excess. If the Liver gets strong

Figure 19. Liver Attacks Spleen And Insults Lungs

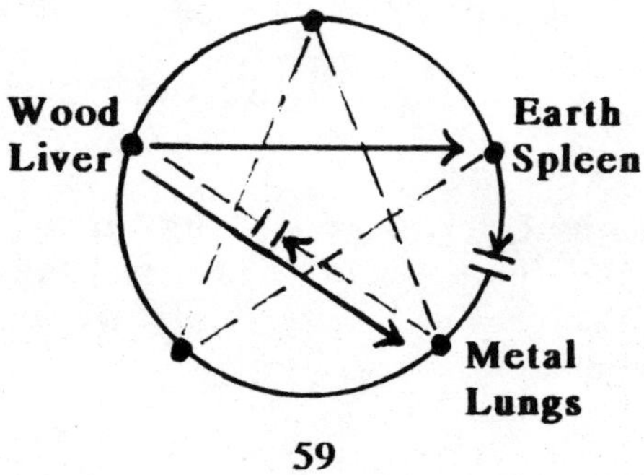

enough and the Lungs weak enough, the Liver may even "insult" the Lungs backwards against the normal flow of the *Ke* cycle. Because the Lungs no longer descend the Qi, the Large Intestine fails to discharge feces and there is constipation. This constipation or Stagnant Qi in the Lower Burner, further congests the Liver which becomes even more Excess.

If the Liver "catches fire" or becomes so Excess as to transform into Heat or Fire, it will suck up all the Yin fuel out of the Kidneys, its mother. This leads to Yin Deficiency of the Kidneys. The ultimate Yin of the Kidneys is the *Jing* Essence. In Chinese medicine, since some *Jing* is required for the creation of new Blood, it is said that the *Jing* and Blood share a common source. This source is the Kidney Yin. Therefore, Kidney Yin Deficiency can lead to Liver Blood Deficiency causing dysmenorrhea, hypomenorrhea, delayed periods, amenorrhea, blurred vision, numbness and tingling of the extremities, photophobia, and Blood Deficiency headache. It can also lead to polyuria, low back pain, and an emptiness of the Sea of Marrow.

Figure 20. Liver Yang exhausting Kidney Yin according to the *Sheng* Cycle.

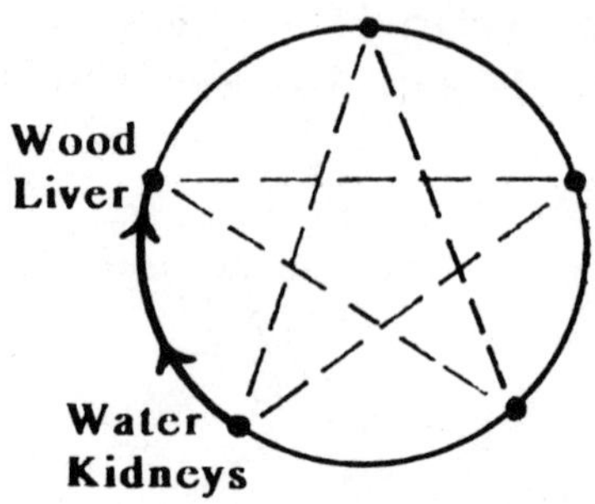

And finally, if the Liver "burns up", its Excessive Heat can be transferred to the Heart. There it can disturb the *Shen* or Spirit-consciousness thus causing anxiety, mental agitation, restlessness, fear, and insomnia.

Figure 21. Transmission of Liver Heat to the Heart according to the *Sheng Cycle*.

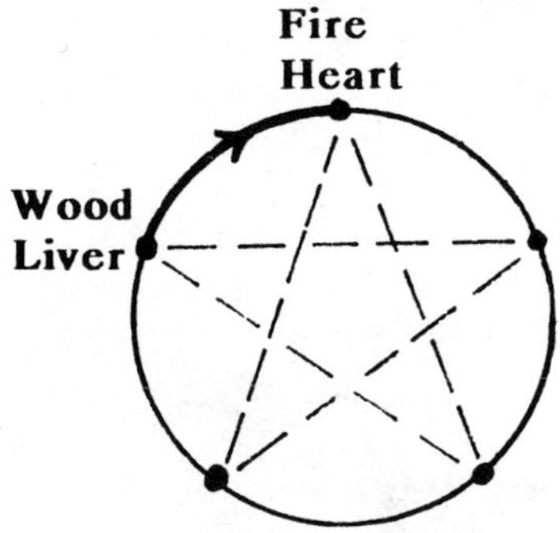

CHINESE THEORY OF MENSTRUATION

Since migraines in women are often associated in some way with their menstrual cycle, it is also necessary to understand something of the Chinese theory of menstruation. And any Chinese discussion of menstruation begins with the Blood.

According to Chinese medical theory, the Blood is created through the interaction of three Organs: the Spleen, Kidneys, and Heart. The Spleen takes the refined Liquid Essence of food and drink and sends this up to the Heart. The Kidneys likewise send up to the Heart some *Jing* Essence. *Jing* Essence is the most primal substance in the body. We are endowed with a certain amount of *Jing* Essence at birth and we also manufacture some from the surplus of energy we don't use day to day. Both Congenital and Acquired Essences are stored in the Kidneys. When the body needs either a quick infusion of energy or the substrate for building new tissue or substance, *Jing* Essence is used. Therefore, the Chinese concept of Blood is created out of the Liquid Essence of food and drink transformed and transported up to the Heart by the Spleen and from *Jing* or Kidney Essence. These the Heart combines to create Blood which the Heart then pumps out to the rest of the body.

Menstrual Blood is relatively excess Blood. It is sent down to the Uterus by the Heart in order to become the source and sustenance of the fetus. Since the Chinese did not use microscopic inspection, traditional Chinese doctors did not know about eggs. They could see the Blood issuing from the vagina and babies too. And they knew men ejaculated sperm into the vagina and that only then did women become pregnant. So throughout Asia it is traditionally believed that the fetus is conceived out of the combination of the woman's Blood and the man's sperm. For a woman to either menstruate or conceive, she must have a superabundance of Blood beyond what is necessary for her own day to day survival.

The *Nei Jing*, the oldest written classic of Chinese medicine, says that women begin to menstruate at fourteen when their Kidneys and their Spleens,i.e. their digestion, have matured, thus creating a monthly superabundance of Blood. According to this view, until fourteen, women's metabolism is not mature and thus does not make sufficient Blood for there to be enough to periodically brim over. The onset of menstruation both at menarche and each month is called the arrival of the *Tian Kui* or Heavenly Water.

In a sense, the Uterus is like a cup. Blood is sent down to the Uterus by the Heart. When the Blood collects sufficiently, it overflows and there is menstruation or the discharge of Blood from the Uterus. In Chinese medicine, the Uterus and the Liver are closely related. In some ways, they are almost synonymous. The Uterus is the Blood Chamber but it is the Liver which stores the Blood. That is one of the Liver's main Chinese medical functions. If the Liver stores properly adequate Blood, menstruation occurs on schedule and is normal in volume.

Another function of the Liver is to maintain patency or free flow of the Qi or vital energy of the body. The Qi and Blood are intimately connected. The Qi moves the Blood and so is its "commander". But the Blood is the Root of the Qi and so is its "mother". If the Qi does not flow smoothly, neither will the Blood. In that case, the Blood will not be able to overflow the Uterus at the proper time nor in the proper amount.

A normal menstrual cycle should span twenty-eight days. Twenty-eight days is also the length of the moon cycle. Therefore, in Chinese, menstruation is called *Yue Jing* or Moon Flow. This twenty-eight day cycle is divided into four seven day segments. The first seven day segment begins with the onset of menstruation and is the menstruation itself. During the menstruation, the Qi or energy mobilizes the Blood for discharge from the uterus and ultimately from the body. The second seven day segment is the postmentruum. During this time, the Blood is relatively Deficient, its surplus having been discharged, and the body is actively engaged in replacing this lost Blood. At the same time, the Qi in the body is travelling upwards and outwards away from the pelvis. It is at this point that the Spleen is sending up the Liquids to be transformed into Blood in and by the Heart. The third segment corresponds to the mid-cycle. At this point, the Blood is relatively full and the Qi starts travelling back down and in, carrying the Blood towards the pelvis. The fourth segment of the cycle is the premenstruum. Here the Qi is attempting to move the Blood to the Uterus in preparation for discharge. At this point, the Qi and Blood are at their maximum volume in the pelvis. Figures 22 and 23 show the important energetic relationships during the four phases of this cycle.

Figure 22. Blood during the 4 phases of a woman's monthly cycle.

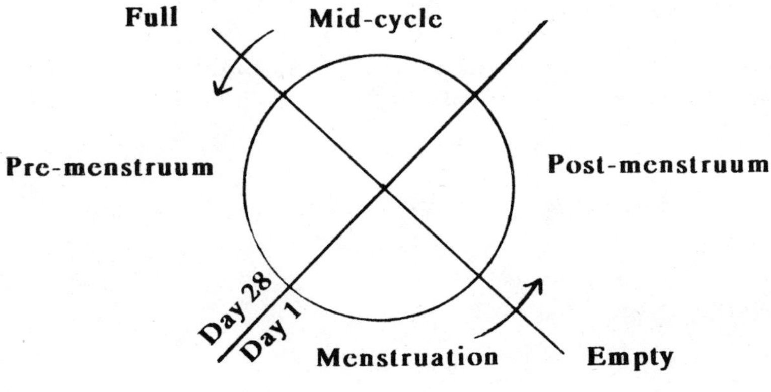

Figure 23. Qi during the 4 phases of a woman's monthly cycle.

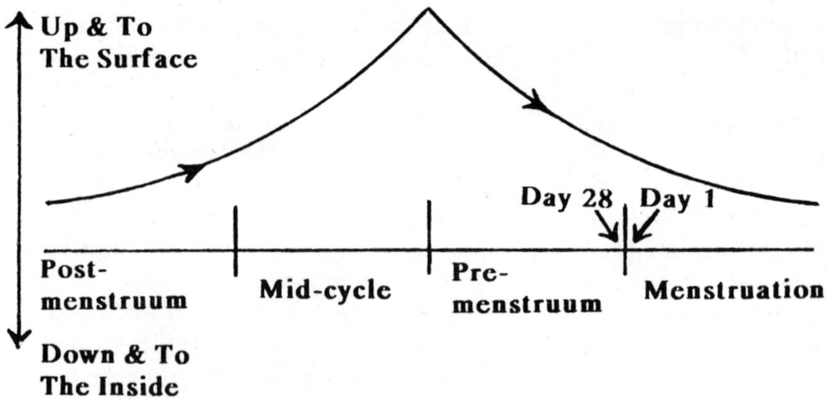

To summarize the above, from the end of menstruation through mid-cycle, the Blood grows in volume. From mid-cycle through menstruation, the Blood flows down and eventually out of the body. The Qi, on the other hand, flows up and to the Surface from the end of menstruation to mid-cycle. From mid-cycle through menstruation, the Qi flows down and in, collecting and then mobilizing the Blood. Because the Qi and Blood are a Yin Yang pair, they are interdependent and their growth and flow depend on each other.

CHINESE DISEASE MECHANISMS FOR THE SIGNS & SYMPTOMS OF MIGRAINES

Traditional Chinese medicine over the last two thousand years has evolved a very complicated energetic physiology or description of how the body works in health and disease. In terms of disease, these *Bing Ji* or disease mechanisms have little to do with the chemical pathophysiology of Western medicine. However, these mechanisms are, nevertheless, logically consistent within themselves and with the whole of Chinese medical theory, and therapy based on these mechanisms has proven itself empirically effective in clinical practice over two millennia. Moreover, these disease mechanisms are understandable on an every day, common sense level. They are based on the direct perception of the natural world of which we are all a part, and they make a kind of immediate sense that the explanations of Western medicine so often do not. In using the theory of Chinese medicine to explain all the various signs and symptoms of migraines, we will basically recapitulate the format of our chapter on "The Western Description of Migraine" attempting to address, point for point, all the idiosyncracies of these headaches.

CLASSICAL MIGRAINE

As stated above, classical migraines start with some visual disturbance. These can be divided basically into two broad categories: 1) seeing what is not normally there, and 2) not seeing what normally is.[90] If the migraineur sees bright lights, is photophobic, or has intense visual hallucinations, this is described in Chinese medicine as an Excess of Yang in the upper part of the body and specifically the head. Yang is associated with light, heat, activity, and upward movement. When Yang energy is Excess, it tends to rise. Since this Yang energy is usually derived from or associated with the Chinese Liver, and since the Liver Meridian travels internally to the eyes, such an upsurge of Yang energy first causes an increase in visual activity. This is based also on the Chinese statement that the eyes are the orifice or window of the Liver.

If, on the other hand, there is tunnel vision, partial blindness, or blurred vision, this is due to Liver Blood Deficiency. It is said in Chinese medicine that the Blood nourishes the Liver and enables the eyes to see. If they are incapable of seeing, this suggests lack of Liver Blood in the head to nourish the eyes and support the visual function. Therefore, this type of visual disturbance is associated with Liver Blood/Kidney Yin Deficiency type migraine. Whereas, the preceding type of visual disturbance is associated with Liver Yang Excess species. In some cases, where there is Liver Yang Excess in combination with Liver Blood/Kidney Yin Deficiency, there may initially be the first type of visual disturbance followed by the second type as the Excess Yang exhausts the Yin in the head.

Another aspect of classical migraines is that they tend to begin on only one side of the head. This is because the Yang energy which rises up out of the Liver is most often shunted into the Gallbladder Channel which is paired with the Liver. The Liver is inherently Yin and often shunts Yang energy into its paired Yang Channel, the Gallbladder Meridian. The Gallbladder Meridian laces the sides of the body and especially criss-crosses the temporal region of the head. Because the Gallbladder Meridian is neither on the back nor the front of the body but on the sides, imbalances in the flow of Qi along this Channel often express themselves as one-sided pathologies.

However, the Yang energy not only moves up but also attempts to disperse outwards towards the Surface. It, therefore, moves into the more superficial Channels and Collaterals which branch from the main Channels. One of these more superficial layers of Channels is called the *Jing Jin* or Channel Sinews. These Channels connect upon the head with the *Jing Jin* branching off of the other main Meridians. Therefore, this Yang energy typically spills over into these other, connected superficial Channels and this explains why the pain of migraine often progresses to encompass the entire head after starting on just one side of the Gallbladder Meridian.

Yet another aspect of a classical migraine is nausea and vomiting. The Liver and Stomach are both closely connected according to Chinese medical theory. When one becomes Excess, so typically will the other. As Excess Liver energy or Yang vents itself upwards, it drafts with it Stomach Qi. This is called, according to Five Phase Theory, Liver invading the Stomach. Stomach Qi is supposed to go down. If its Qi perverts upwards, this is experienced as nausea and potentially vomiting. If a migraine episode is terminated by vomiting, it is because, in the act of vomiting, Stomach Qi is dispersed or discharged. This reduction in Stomach Qi then mutually reduces the closely connected Liver Qi, thus reducing the Excess Yang jamming upwards into the head.

If the Spleen is also weak, the Liver may also invade it. This is called *Gan Fan Pi*, Liver invading the Spleen. This results in the Spleen becoming Deficient. Spleen Qi is supposed to travel upwards. If it becomes too weak, it falls downward. This diminution in Spleen Qi also causes fatigue and chilling since the Spleen is the so-called Postnatal Root of energy and, therefore, warmth production. Some migraines end in voiding of the stools or diarrhea. This is due to weakening of the Spleen, and the diarrhea is an expression of the Spleen Qi's falling downwards. Since the Spleen Qi is the Root of Postnatal Qi, including the Qi of the Liver, if it becomes too weak, this also weakens the Stomach and Liver Qi, thus also reducing their Excess. When this happens, the patient is left extremely weak and fatigues at the end of their headache.

The length of time between classical migraines is largely dependent upon how long it takes for the individual to accumulate enough Stagnant Liver Qi before it accumulates to such a point where it has to vent itself somewhere, usually upwards. Since the Qi moves the food through the alimentary canal and also moves Body Fluids, this Qi Stagnation also explains the constipation and oliguria that often precede a migraine. Then, when the Qi vents upwards, the Stagnation vis a vis digestion and urination is relaxed, and, therefore, defecation and urination are often associated with the climax of an attack.

COMMON MIGRAINE

Common migraines are not preceded by any visual disturbance, nor are there any other particular prodromal signs and symptoms. This is because common migraines tend not to be so severe as classical migraines. People with common migraines tend to have more frequent headaches and so Stagnant Qi vents itself upwards much sooner and, therefore, with less force. The disease mechanism does usually still involve upward perversion of Stagnant Liver Qi, and, therefore, the Gallbladder Channel is often involved and the Stomach/Spleen to some, although usually lesser degree. The fact that frequent, periodic, common migraines tend to occur more often in the late hours of the night and early hours of the morning is due to the fact that, according to Chinese medicine, the Gallbladder Channel is at high tide from 11 PM to 1 AM and the Liver Channel from 1 AM to 3 PM. Since these are the times within the diurnal cycle when the Liver and Gallbladder naturally are most Excess, these are the most likely times for these Organs to manifest that Excess even more, similar to high tide occurring simultaneously with a full moon.

That 44% of common migraines are temporal, one-sided headaches attests to the pivotal role of the Liver/Gallbladder in the migraine mechanism. The 22% that experience the headache all over the head are mostly those persons with a chronic Excess in the *Jing Jin* in the upper part of their body. This is due to a chronic plethora of Yang above. The 14% who experience bilateral frontal headaches are those whose headache has to do with the Liver's relationship to the Stomach and Large Intestine more than the Liver's relationship to the Gallbladder. The forehead is the zone of the head irrigated by the *Yang Ming* or Stomach/Large Intestine Channels. The 13% experiencing a one-sided frontal headache are also experiencing pain and Excess in their Gallbladder Meridian stemming from the Liver. The Gallbladder Channel comes to a point just above the eye. For whatever reason, their Qi is primarily stuck and accumulating at this point on the Gallbladder Meridian. The 6% with occipital headaches are either experiencing blockage in the neck portion of their Gallbladder Channels or blockage in their Bladder Channels due to Kidney Yin Deficiency. The Kidney and Bladder Channels have a similar Yin Yang relationship to the Liver/Gallbladder. If the Kidney Yin becomes Deficient, this allows Yang to float upwards along the path of the Bladder Channel to the occiput. And finally, the 1% who experience pain at their vertex are experiencing the final, upward, internal termination of the Liver Channel itself. The Liver Channel comes to and ends at the very crown of the head, and pain at the vertex is due most often to an Excess within the Liver Meridian that has not been shunted into the Gallbladder Channel.

CLUSTER HEADACHE

Cluster headaches most often have to do with Heat and Excess of the Stomach aggravated by Liver Qi. The Stomach Channel comes through the sinuses and irrigates, in part, the nose. Men tend to have cluster headaches more than women because their Stomachs tend to be Hotter and more Excess. Upward perversion of Stomach Qi along the course of the Stomach Meridian thus explains the watery eyes, nasal discharge, sinus pressure, and even epistaxis which often precede or accompany cluster headaches. This perverse Stomach Qi can draft upward either Body Fluids (nasal discharge & watery eyes) or Blood (nosebleed & red eyes). Photophobia is also due to this upward perversion of Yang energy up the Stomach Channel. In particular, the pain is one-sided and periodic because this perverse Qi tends to shunt into another superficial branch of the main Stomach Meridian called the Longitudinal *Luo* or Collateral. *Luo* problems are often one-sided and biorhythmic diurnally.

The periodicity of cluster headaches is related to the periodicity of the Channels and Organs which Chinese medicine describes. This part of Chinese medical theory or biorhythmic theory is called in Chinese *Wu Yun Liu Qi* or the Five Transports/Six Qi. This very profound theory describes in a predictable way all the various hourly, daily, monthly, seasonal, and yearly cycles at work in the body. These are all too complicated and too numerous to describe in this book. However, the fact that most cluster headaches occur in the spring is due to the fact that the Liver is at high tide annually each spring and the Qi of the body is naturally rising upwards longitudinally during this season.

DIVERSITY OF MIGRAINE SIGNS & SYMPTOMS

That migraineurs experience a wide variety of signs and symptoms is due to the fact that there is no single mechanism for migraine, although the Liver usually does play its part. In fact, there are as many complicated disease mechanism scenarios for migraine as there are migraine sufferers. Since each person's constitution and condition is different and ever changing, so each person's energetic physiology is also variable. Nonetheless, we can describe the most common disease mechanisms for the most common signs and symptoms accompanying migraines.

We have already discussed visual disturbances, hallucinations, nausea, and vomiting. Dizziness can be due to either an Excess of Yang Qi pounding upwards into and disturbing the head or a Deficiency of Blood or Yin. The professional practitioner is capable of distinguishing these two, diametrically opposite disease mechanisms based on subtle differences in their felt experience. Numbness is usually due to Blood Deficiency; whereas, tingling may be due to Internal Stirring of Wind, i.e. erratic movement of the Qi either due to Blood Deficiency or Excess Yang Qi. Tension is due to Stagnant Qi and detachment or temporary withdrawal is also usually due to failure of the Qi to circulate outward from the inside. Depression and irritability are likewise due to Depressive Liver Qi. Yawning is either an attempt to liberate Stagnant Qi or an effort to recoup Deficient Qi.

Hunger as part of a migraine attack suggests an over-heated Stomach. Talkativeness is due to Yang energy rising to the upper part of the body in general and Heat accumulating in the Heart in particular, since, according to Chinese medical theory, speech is largely a reflection of that Organ. Whereas, loss of memory for words and names is usually due to Liver Blood Deficiency/Kidney

Yin Deficiency. Slurred speech and incoherence can be either due to Qi Deficiency, in which case the person doesn't have the energy to articulate, or due to Heat again collecting in the Heat having risen up out of the Liver/Stomach. Trembling and tremor are manifestations of Stirring of Internal Wind. This Wind is Qi which is running wild. Mild tremors may be due to insufficient Blood and Yin to hold the Qi in place. More violent tremors and spasticity suggest Excess Yang or Liver Fire venting themselves after having accumulated under pressure.

We have already discussed the Chinese mechanisms for pain. Skin rash accompanying migraines are usually due to Heat in the Liver over-heating the Blood. The Liver stores the Blood according to Chinese medicine, and Heat in the Liver can easily be transferred to the Blood. The Blood then 'boils' up and over towards the Surface, where it manifests as a rash. If, on the other hand, there are hives, these are due to Internal Wind blowing to the surface. Swelling of the fingers, hands, wrists, ankles, and legs is due to the Spleen's inability to transport and transform Liquids in turn due to that Organ's being over-controlled by and Excess Liver. Whereas, a swollen lower abdomen and breasts are a direct manifestation of Liver Qi Stagnation. This Qi accumulates in any area traversed by the Liver Channel, and, in women, the hypogastrium and breasts are prime targets, especially with menstrually related migraines.

Inability to concentrate is usually due to either weak Spleen function in turn due to Liver Excess or Heat rising up from the Liver and Stomach accumulating in the Heart. In the first case, there is not enough Qi to think, and in the second, the Spirit or *Shen*, i.e. the consciousness, is disturbed by the Heat and, therefore, has a tendency to flit about. Constipation accompanying migraines is due to Liver Qi Stagnation causing Large Intestine Stagnation as well. It is the free flow of the Liver Qi which insures the free flow of peristalsis. Diarrhea, on the other hand, is most often due to weak or Deficient Spleen Qi. As mentioned above, often these two symptoms alternate during a migrainous attack, constipation preceding the attack and diarrhea occurring at its denouement. Also as mentioned above, decreased urination is due to Liver Qi's retarding Liquid transportation; whereas increased urination is either the result of the Liver Qi having vented itself or of an over-heated Stomach. When the Stomach gets Hot, it often over-transports Water downwards. This is called "Side-tracking of Fluids" in Chinese medicine. Also in Chinese medicine it is said, the Kidneys are the sluice-gate of the Stomach.

MENSTRUAL MIGRAINE

There are two basic kinds of menstrual migraines according to Chinese medicine. Most premenstrual migraines are due to the accumulation of Qi and Blood in the Liver which occurs from mid-cycle to the onset of menstruation. This aggravates any pre-existing Excess in the Liver of either Stagnant Qi or Heat. This Stagnant Qi and Heat transform into Yang which vents itself upwards along the Liver or Gallbladder Meridians. Such premenstrual Excess migraines are of the Liver Fire, Liver Wind, Ascension of Liver Yang variety. Their pain is usually abrupt and severe.

Postmenstrual migraines or migraines which occur at or towards the end of the period are due more to Deficiency. A certain amount of Blood is lost during the period. This may leave insuficient Blood to "fill up" the body and nourish the Brain. This type of migraine is usually more insidious and drawn-out. Essentially, there is not enough Blood in the upper body to maintain patency of flow in the head.
Many women have a combination of both these two basic types of menstrual migraine. They have Excess Liver Qi and Heat *and* Deficient Spleens and Blood. The Blood accumulates in the pelvis below, but the Qi may "separate" from the Blood and flush back upwards toward the head. This may cause migraines, tension headaches, palpitations, breast swelling and pain, and emotional hypersensitivity. This up-flush of Qi from the pelvis is the classical origin of the word hysteria, *hystero* meaning womb in Greek. In nineteenth century Western medicine, it was called "the vapors". Women with such combination migraines have a combination of both Excess and Deficiency signs and symptoms.

Migraines often stop during pregnancy because whatever Excesses there are in terms of Qi and Blood are made use of in nourishing the fetus. In addition, the energetic circulation from the Heart to

Kidneys at the core of the body is strongly directed down towards the womb, and the fetus tends to act as a root for the woman's Yang, the fetus' body being Yin.

HEMIPLEGIC MIGRAINE

The signs and symptoms of hemiplegic migraine share essentially the same disease mechanism in Chinese medicine as stroke or what used to be known as apoplexy. Liver Qi Stagnation accumulates until there is enough internal pressure that it vents itself upwards as Wind along the Gallbladder Meridian. This Wind drafts with it Phlegm which can lodge in the Channel and Collaterals causing loss of feeling and movement due to its obstructing the passage of Qi and Blood. It is the Qi which empowers movement and the Blood which enables sensation. In Chinese medicine, uprushing Qi causing hemiplegia is called *Zhong Feng*, Penetrating Wind.

OPHTHALMOPLEGIC MIGRAINE

This relatively rare species of migraine is also due to the same mechanism described above, *Zhong Feng*. However, in this case, the Liver Qi remains within the Liver Meridian instead of being shunted in the Gallbladder Channel. It drafts with it Phlegm and this Phlegm obstructs the internal course of the Liver Meridian connecting directly with the eyes. Loss of movement and even loss of vision are again due to obstruction by Phlegm of the Qi and Blood respectively.

FACIAL MIGRAINE

In my experience, facial migraines are usually due to a combination of Liver Qi and Heat mixed with Kidney Yin Deficiency. The teeth are an outgrowth of the Kidneys according to Chinese medicine, and chronic, recurrent pain in the cheeks and teeth is usually due to Deficiency Fire Flaring Upward. This is most often encountered in elderly patients with a previous history of common or classical migraines who are not robust enough to generate that much internal pressure any more. Photophobia and phonophobia in such patients are also due to Yin Deficiency. The Yin insures the capacity of the sense organs to function. When Yin is insufficient, the sense organs may be overwhelmed by their stimuli, thus leading to photophobia (Liver Blood) and phonophobia (Kidney Yin).

BASILAR MIGRAINE

The fact that it is mostly teenage girls who get this rare form of migraine is due to its disease mechanism being associated in Chinese medicine with what is called the arrival of the *Tian Kui*. *Tian Kui* means Heavenly Water and saying that the Heavenly Water has arrived is a poetic way of referring to menarche. The Heaven in this compound therm refers to the Heart and upper half of the body which must send down sufficient Blood for there to be enough to overflow the Uterus on a monthly basis. The Water in this term refers to Kidney Water or Kidney Yin which also irrigates the Uterus and supplies it with *Jing* Essence, a constituent of the Blood. In some young women who are Yin Deficient, the period leaves the Heart Blood and Yin Deficient and the Kidneys Yin Deficient as well. Deficiency Fire flares up to disturb the *Shen* in the Heart causing incoherent speech, slurred speech, fainting, giddiness, and visual disturbance. The pain is experienced at the base of the skull or occiput because, similar to the Liver venting Yang Qi into the Gallbladder Channel, Kidney Yang energy tends to flare up the associated Bladder Meridian, it being Yang compared to the Kidney Meridian being Yin.

MIGRAINE EQUIVALENTS

Migraine equivalents describe a large number of signs and symptoms which often are associated with migraine headaches but also may present on their own without head pain. Western medicine is correct in intuiting a connection between these signs and symptoms and migraine, but it is Chinese medical theory which really explains their mechanisms and precise relationships.

For instance, many persons experience the prodromal signs and symptoms of migraine without this leading necessarily to head pain. This can include visual disturbances or displays and numbness and tingling. In such cases, there is sufficient Liver Qi accumulated to vent itself upwards and outwards but insufficient Qi to cause obstruction and pain in the head. Although the Yang

Qi is more than usual, it still can be accommodated by cephalic circulation so that it does not cause pressure and pain.

Periodic vomiting and bilious attacks are often due to Stagnant Liver Qi venting itself into the Stomach. In Chinese, this is called *Gan Fan Wei*, Liver attacking the Stomach. Likewise, this can also cause abdominal pain and epigastric bloating. If, however, the Liver invades or attacks the Spleen, this typically causes diarrhea. The Liver is Excess and the Spleen is Deficient. The Spleen cannot transport and transform foods and liquids properly and so diarrhea ensues. Precordial or pseudoangina migraine is called Heart or Chest *Bi* in Chinese. Thus means obstruction in the Heart or chest due to Qi Stagnation. All three of these scenarios -- Liver invading Stomach, Liver invading Spleen, and Liver causing Chest *Bi* -- are common stress reactions. Depending upon the individual constitution and disposition, some people will experience certain of these reactions at certain biorhythmic times or due to certain types of stimuli.

In fact, that any of these so-called migraine equivalents can alternate with true migraines, either common or classic, underscores the fact that migraines are not a single disease in the same way that polio or scarlatina are. Rather, migraines and all their associated and alternate signs and symptoms are manifestations of imbalance in a number of Organs and Bowels -- primarily the Liver, Gallbladder, Spleen, and Stomach. Depending upon stress, diet, lifestyle, sex, season, weather, temperature, phase of the moon, and an infinite other stimuli and variables, the pathologic relationships between these various Organs, Bowels, and Body Humors may manifest in multifarious ways. Happily, traditional Chinese medical theory can make clear and rational sense of all the whys and wherefores of these variations on a theme.

As Western clinicians have noted for hundreds, if not thousands of years, migraines are a species of stress reaction. Almost always there is some degree of Liver Qi Stagnation at the root of migraines and their equivalents. In the past, both Western and Oriental clinicians described a migraine personality and their descriptions were virtually identical. However, today, stress in the modern world is so pervasive and endemic that we no longer can isolate a migraine personality. In a sense, modern life has made us all migraine personalities, since almost every adult American has some clinically identifiable amount of Liver Qi in their Chinese energetic diagnosis.

The fact that migraineurs are prone to certain other health disorders underscores the fact that Liver Qi is the underlying disease mechanism for the majority of these related conditions. There are several different disease mechanisms for each of ulcerative colitis, psoriasis, hayfever, asthma, urticaria, Meniere's disease, peptic ulcer, Crohn's disease, nightmares, PMS, constipation, diarrhea, tension headaches, functional heart disease, essential hypertension, rhinitis, upper respiratory infections, psychoneuroses, and motion sickness, *but the one disease mechanism which is common to all of these is Liver Qi.*

THE NATURAL HISTORY OF MIGRAINES

As described above, Dr. Sacks divides the course of a single migrainous attack into five stages. Chinese medical theory also has a clear description of the energetic mechanisms at work during each of these stages.

Excitation

The initial excitation stage is the period where Stagnant Liver Qi is building to a definite, pathological Excess. Qi in Chinese medicine is function and Qi and the mind are seen as two aspects of a single reality. Therefore, as the Qi becomes Excess, we experience states of excitation and arousal, i.e. hyperfunction: hyeracusis, hypersensitivity, visual arousal, and tingling. This accumulation of Qi may be experienced as depression if the Liver Qi is, in a Chinese medical sense, Depressed, or it may be experienced as elation as the first Qi begins to vent upwards. This Excess of Qi, which is inherently Yang in Chinese philosophic terms, may also lead to restlessness and insomnia and even altered states of consciousness, such as *deja vu* and *jamais vu*.

That the initial attack seems to come out of nowhere or is sudden in onset is due to the Qi having accumulated slowly, slowly to a point of no return. An internal balance is tipped and a process is suddenly put in motion. Since the various stimuli generating this process are so numerous, it may seem like the process lacks a definite stimulus. However, the stimuli are often a multitude of microtraumata or small insults to the system rather than just one big, obvious one.

The compelling quality of the experience is due to the fact that we are experiencing a gush of Qi or Wind venting itself up the core of our beings. In Oriental medicine, the Qi and the mind are sometimes likened to a horse and rider. In this case, the horse or Qi is running off with the mind and is out of conscious control. At root, the Qi and mind are identical, even though we normally assume there is an I somewhere within which is separate and distinct and in control. Like many climatic life events, such as birth and birthing and death itself, migraines show the error of this illusion.

The timeless quality of this experience or out of time sense is also an aspect of this experience's interrupting our normal, habitual mental patterns. Past, present, and future are likewise artificial contrivances of the thinking mind which are interrupted by this swoosh of upward venting Qi. This experience is so intense and so interrupts our usual, everyday mode of thinking, that for a brief period, we come close to experiencing our mind itself as opposed to its various thought displays. Throughout time, all humans have failed to find words to convey this preconceptual state.

Engorgement

During the engorgement phase, so much Qi and Blood have risen into the upper or cephalic part of the body, they cannot flow freely. The skull is a closed box which can only accommodate so much Qi and Blood without obstruction and pressure. As an Excess of Qi and Blood accumulates in the head, so the pain increases. As we have already seen, where the pain is felt depends upon which Meridian or Meridians are the most jammed and obstructed. This jamming is concurrently experienced as muscular tension (especially in the neck which is exactly a bottleneck), constipation, decreased urination, irritability, restlessness, and an inability to accept any further Qi into the system, whether that be sight, sound, touch, or smell.

Prostration

The prostration stage is evidence that the Qi which has vented itself upwards have been expended and discharged. The patient's Righteous Qi is exhausted below and they experience lethargy, fatigue, and lassitude. They have no energy left to do anything, to communicate, to be active. They are literally energetically spent like an empty shell casing after the bullet has been fired.

Resolution

The attack may be resolved either by falling asleep or by some metabolic discharge which causes a release of Qi and thus pulls the rug right out from under the swoosh of up-rushing Qi. Such releases of Qi may be physical or emotional, but all result in a discharge of Qi, thus bleeding off the source of the attack. Physical discharges causing diminution of Qi include sex, urination, defecation, vomiting, and sweating. Emotional discharges include crying, screaming, venting of rage, or the expression of any strong emotion. Physical activity can also bleed off the Qi as well. Vomiting is the most common discharge putting an end to migraines. Stomach Qi is discharged with vomiting, and since the Stomach is the Root of so much Qi in the body, vomiting reduces the total Qi of the body to such an extent that the state of Excess flips to Deficiency.

Rebound

Rebound describes the phase where the person's Qi returns to a normal, healthy level. It has not yet accumulated to its chronic pathological level, and so the person feels even better than normal, normal here meaning somewhat malaised. The person experiences abundance of Qi without Stagnation -- real health, even if it is only temporary.

PERIODICITY

The fact that 43% of migraineurs develop their first migraines between the ages of 11 and 20 is due to the fact that during puberty the *Ming Men Zhi Huo* or the Fire of the Gate of Life reaches maturity. This Fire is the Root of all warmth in the organism. It is associated with the Kidney Yang and it is relatively immature until the early teens. Most of the health complaints of teenagers, such as acne and behavioral difficulties, are due to this *Ming Men* Fire's "kicking in". This Fire is the basis of sexual Fire, but it also provides the warmth for the Stomach, Spleen, Liver, Gallbladder, and Heart/Pericardium as well. All these Organs participate in the *Ming Men*, and if any one of these becomes over-heated, any or all of the others may also become Excess. Most typically, this Excess manifests in disturbances of the Stomach and Liver, Stomach Heat giving rise to acne and insatiable appetite, and Liver Heat giving rise to anger, frustration, and depression. Also during the teenage years, there are increased mental and emotional stresses, social, sexual, academic, familial, which tend to cause Liver Qi Stagnation. The teenager is somewhat stuck between two phases of life, childhood and adulthood, and this creates internal pressure which, in a Chinese medical sense, accumulates primarily in the Liver. In many people, this Stagnant Qi and Heat vent themselves in an upward rush through the core to be experienced as migraine. In this sense, migraines are one of the body's coping mechanisms. When they are due to Excess, they are like a release valve allowing trapped and pressurized Qi to escape from the torso upwards and outwards.

The nausea and recurrent stomachaches which some children experience before puberty, and especially children who go on to develop migraines, are a venting of this pent-up Qi into the Stomach via the Five Phase Control cycle. During prepubescence, the child may have developed enough stress and, therefore, Liver Qi to require venting, but is not yet Hot enough to build up sufficient pressure for this Qi to blow upwards like a volcano. This also explains the relationship of childhood "bilious attacks" and motion sickness to teenage and young adult migraines.

Infantile eczema as a precursor to the development of migraines has to do with so-called Fetal Toxins or *Tai Du*. This is inherited Heat passed on to the developing fetus either at conception from either parent or during gestation from the mother. This pathologic Heat can be caused by emotional stress, faulty diet, and/or a Hot disease suffered by either parent within a certain time of conception or during gestation by the mother. This Toxic Heat predisposes the child to run too Hot in general. This Heat resides in the *Xue Fen* or Blood level of energy in the child and the Blood is stored in the Liver. Therefore, such Fetal Toxins can predispose specifically the Liver to being over-heated, and it should already by clear how an over-heated Liver predisposes a person to migraine.

The fact that migraines tend to get better with age can be explained by several different mechanisms according to Chinese medicine. First, the *Ming Men* declines with age and the Qi and Blood naturally become Deficient. This natural decline causes a diminution in Heat and in Qi Stagnation. There is just not enough Heat and Qi for the person to continue building such internal pressure. In some cases, patients may report a history of migraines throughout their teenage and adult years. Then they may report a "cessation" of migraines with advancing age, only to be, in fact, suffering from facial migraines which they do not recognize as the same basic phenomenon. The difference is that when the person was robust, they experienced cataclysmic upheaval, but now they are more like a perpetually smoldering volcano. This is the difference between an up-flushing Excess and an upward flaring Deficiency.

Women who experience menstrual migraines often report a cessation of migraines with menopause. In this case, the woman's Blood has become exhausted to the point where she cannot support any longer a monthly discharge of Blood. The body, in its homeostatic wisdom, therefore, shuts off the menstruation. However, since the Blood is the mother of the Qi, the woman's Liver becomes Deficient in general along with the Kidneys which are its foundation or root. Although she may still experience pent-up Qi due to stress, there again is not enough Qi to vent explosively upwards.

Other women experience the onset of migraines or an aggravation of migraines at menopause. In these women, because of Deficiency of Yin due to age, their Yang flares up into the upper part of the body. This can cause a temporary relative Excess of Liver Yang in the upper body. This Excess may last several months or several years, but since its root has been cut, i.e. Liver Blood/Kidney Yin, eventually it too becomes exhausted. Women who get migraines at menopause are relatively more robust than those whose migraines disappear at menopause. Parenthetically, hot flashes are also a species of up-flushing Yang energy from the Liver and Kidneys.

Another factor leading to the cessation of migraines with age, and one which should not be over-looked, is that many older persons have less stress in their lives. They may not be working so much or so hard. Their children are established on their own. Their careers are over or they are now reaping the rewards of a lifetime of hard work. They may also have learned the lessons of life and are thus able to cope better with themselves within and the world without. In other words, they may have finally learned how to relax and keep things in proper perspective.

Periodic migraines are those which occur on a fixed schedule irrespective of lifestyle and diet. Various individuals will have migraine episodes at different frequencies depending on various factors. Weekly migraines most often occur on weekends. In such cases, the patient has managed to keep their pent-up Qi under control throughout the week. But then, when they can relax and do, this pent-up Liver Qi flushes upwards. To some, this seems paradoxical, but to the Chinese doctor, it seems quite obvious.

Other periodic migraines are more clearly associated with large micro-macrocosmic rhythms. For instance, on a monthly basis, the volume of the Qi grows with the waxing of the moon and travels upwards longitudinally in the body. If a person's Liver Qi is pent-up already, it will be under more pressure whenever the Qi is fuller in general, and it will be all the more likely to vent itself upward if the Qi flow in general is upward. This also explains annual migraines occurring in the spring, which, according to Chinese medicine, runs for 72 days after the first week in February. At this time too, the volume of Qi is growing and is also moving up globally in the body. Full moons in spring are, then, especially potent periods for the exacerbation of migraines. Those persons who suffer migraines at the new moon, on the other hand, tend to have Blood Deficiency migraines.

Once the pent-up Qi has vented itself and is spent, it takes time for this Qi to build up again to sufficient pressure to again "pop off". Therefore, those persons whose migraines are primarily aggravated by biorhythmic or macrocosmic periodicity experience a grace period during which there is insufficient Qi accumulated to vent itself no matter what the lifestyle or dietary stimuli. However, once the Qi has accumulated sufficiently, depending upon the constitution and condition of the individual, any number of stimuli may set off the attack within a certain time range, and, even without any overt stimulus, the Qi may simply reach its own internal limit of pressure and compaction.

EPIDEMIOLOGY

The fact that twice as many women get migraines as men is explained by the fact that migraines are primarily associated with Chinese Liver dysfunction and menstruation is also largely controlled by the Liver. In Chinese medicine, the Kidneys are called the Prenatal Organ in men, but the Liver is pre-eminent in women. In addition, I think it is fair to say that women experience more stress and frustration then men without the same avenues for that stress' release and discharge. Therefore, the higher incidence of migraines in women is both physiological and sociological.

The fact that migraines run in families is more likely due to shared emotional experience and learned emotional coping behavior. There is no theory of Congenital Liver Qi Stagnation in traditional Chinese medicine, although there are other congenital diseases it does describe. Some individuals are Hotter than others and have more Qi and Blood, but Stagnant Qi is not communicated through the sperm and egg (or Blood in traditional Chinese medicine). That is not to say, however, that an individual may not be karmically predisposed to migraines on an esoteric level.

THE CAUSES OF MIGRAINES

EMOTIONS

As discussed above, the first set of migraine stimuli are emotional factors. Chinese medicine says that any frustration, whether physical, mental, or emotional may cause Stagnant Qi. Further, Stagnant Qi is experienced as irritability, temper, anger, and depression. These emotions are an expression of Stagnant Qi but also further aggravate and perpetuate Stagnant Qi. As Dr. Sacks also points out, all violent emotions tend to "arrest a person in mid-excitement or immediately following the peak of excitement."[91] This arrest in the flow of experience is nothing other than an arrest in the flow of Qi. Dr. Sacks goes on to say that many migraineurs are caught in a mental-emotional "bind" and this is exactly what the Chinese concept of Qi Stagnation describes on an energetic level. When the Qi cannot flow freely, it backs up and accumulates. When it accumulates to the limits of the person's capacity to hold it in check, it vents itself somewhere, either violently or not, either up, down, laterally, or to the Surface. In the case of migraineurs, it usually vents itself upwards.

EXHAUSTION, EXERCISE, & SEX

Extreme exhaustion can trigger a migraine in either of two ways. One, it can cause consumption of Blood which often is insufficient to either hold the Qi down or to nourish and keep open the pathways of the head. Or two, fatigue can cause a relaxation of pent-up Qi internally. It takes Qi to hold on to Qi, and if the holding Qi becomes exhausted, the held Qi may escape.

Exercise is one way to vent pent-up Qi. Usually it is one of the best voluntary antidotes to the involuntary venting of migraines. However, in some cases, exercise may mobilize pent-up Qi, but, before it can circulate and bleed off this Qi, the Qi rushes upwards out of control. Exercise itself first causes an increase in internal pressure which is only subsequently followed by a decrease. If the Qi is close to "blowing its cork" in any case, exercise may push this pressure over the edge before it has a chance to dissipate it.

We have already discussed the relationship of the *Ming Men* Fire to the Liver. Therefore, it should come as no surprise that sex can initiate a migraine or that migraines can be accompanied by sexual arousal. Sex inflames the *Ming Men* and thus the Liver, but, conversely, Liver Heat can also inflame the *Ming Men* thus giving rise to sexual arousal. Orgasm is a crescendo of Yang energy released from the pelvis or Lower Burner. In some people, orgasm can bleed off an impending migraine; in other people or at other times, it can push this pent-up Yang Qi over the edge and make its venting and upward discharge all the more violent or likely.

IRREGULAR MEALS

Skipping meals or eating at irregular intervals may provoke migraines in certain individuals. Usually, in Chinese medicine, these are persons with weak Spleen Qi. According to Five Phase Theory, the Liver keeps the Spleen in check, but a strong, healthy Spleen can also keep the Liver in check. Missing meals and fasting weakens the Spleen, especially in persons who would be described as hypoglycemic from the Western point of view. This decline in Spleen Qi thus allows the Liver to blow upwards, in Chinese medicine it being the Spleen Qi which "holds" or restrains everything in the body.

ALCOHOL

Alcohol is described as being Hot and Damp and "enters" or goes to the Liver in Chinese medicine. Because it enters the Liver, it makes the Liver Hot. Because it is Damp, it makes the Spleen weak. As we have already seen, a Hot Liver and a Damp Spleen are a good recipe for a migraine. In addition, alcohol is outwardly and upwardly dispersing according to Chinese medicine and, therefore, can directly precipitate the venting of Liver Qi. This is exactly why we like to drink when we are up-tight. However, if we are too tightly wrapped, this immediate mobilization and relaxation may result in violent upward discharge in persons prone to migraines

SMOKING

Likewise, nicotine is also dispersing and discharging and can precipitate the venting of pent-up Liver Qi. And again, this is also why people smoke, to relax and bleed off this Qi. Unfortunately, both smoking and drinking can be the trigger setting off the volcano, and, in any case, are not healthy ways to remedy pent-up stress.

PRECIPITATING FOODS

Although different foods may precipitate migraines in different individuals, each of the commonly listed aggravating foods can be explained by Chinese medical theory.

Chocolate inflames the *Ming Men* Fire. Its oils and fats dampen the Spleen and cause Excessive Heat in the Stomach and Liver. And its sugar also causes Dampness and weakness of the Spleen. Therefore, it will precipitate migraines in persons with Liver Qi, a Hot Stomach and strong *Ming Men*, and a Damp, Deficient Spleen.

Cheese and milk products are considered Damp and Phlegmatic in Chinese medicine. Milk products tend to aggravate Dampness and weakness of the Spleen at the same time as plugging the Qi pathways with Phlegm. This Phlegm can add to the pressure in the Qi flow system, thus increasing internal pressure and any tendency to Liver Qi Stagnation.

Citrus fruits are also considered extremely dampening in Chinese medicine. They likewise impede Spleen function and, if they contribute to Phlegm production, also aggravate Liver Qi. Many tropical fruits are Cold and thus weaken the Spleen; however, because citrus fruits are Sour and Sour is the flavor which "enters" or goes directly to the Liver and which also causes astringency or tightening, citrus fruits also can cause a marked increase in Liver Qi. Interestingly, Chinese medicine uses several different types of citrus peel to eliminate Dampness and regulate the Qi, thus showing the tendency in nature toward balance and self-correction.

Red wine is not only alcohol but it too is extremely Sour. It has a definite adverse effect on the Liver and contributes to Chinese concepts of Liver disease.

Vegetables are one of our healthiest food groups. However, the Brassica or cabbage/collards family does have carminative properties. Carminatives are medicinal substances which cause flow of pent-up intestinal gas. They do this by pushing the gas out of the body. In Chinese medicine, gas is pent-up Qi or *Zhuo Qi*, Turbid Qi. If Qi is pent-up in the Liver and it is "pushed" by such carminative foods, rather than venting down through the intestines, it may erupt upwards causing migraines. Therefore, persons with Chinese Liver Qi and a tendency to migraines should not eat too much cabbage and its relatives.

Tea and coffee are both used during migraines to relieve the pain. Yet either of these can also trigger an attack. Both are dispersing and discharging according to Chinese medicine, somewhat similar to nicotine and alcohol. Because they are dispersing and discharging, they can discharge pent-up Qi on the verge of erupting. This also explains why persons with Liver Qi often are habituated to tea and coffee. Coffee, in particular, tends to waste or exhaust the Blood and, therefore, also contributes to Blood and Yin Deficiency migraines as well.

Meat tends to be both Hot and Damp according to Chinese medicine. Pork is especially greasy and, therefore, Damp. If a person is over-heated and Damp as well, this can aggravate Hot Liver Qi and precipitate an attack. If the Dampness, Heat, and Qi spread laterally, the person may experience a gallbladder attack or kidney stones. But, if the Dampness, Heat, and Qi vent upwards, this can cause a migraine.

Shellfish, such as mussels and oysters tonify or make strong the Liver and Kidneys. That is great as long as this increase in Qi and Blood can circulate freely. If it cannot, however, it may transform into Heat and vent or flare upwards. Shrimp, on the other hand, cause Heat in the Blood which likewise can be transferred to the Liver.

Depending upon an individual's immediate internal condition, a food listed above may or may not trigger a migraine; or, may trigger a migraine at certain times, but not at others. Whether a food precipitates a migraine attack depends on how that food effects a certain person at a certain time. However, all the foods listed above do fall into clear groupings of dietary mechanisms associated with migraines.

CHANGES IN SLEEP/WAKE CYCLE

As we have seen above, fatigue may cause a release in the holding in of pent-up Liver Qi. Fatigue weakens the Spleen which then allows the Liver to run amok. On the other hand, when we sleep, the Blood returns from the four limbs to be stored in the Liver. This makes the Liver all the more Excess. This return and stasis of Liver Blood may trigger a crescendo of upwardly venting Liver Qi, i.e. a migraine. In addition, a repetitive but relaxed schedule reinforces regular and, therefore, patent Qi flow. Whereas, changes in schedule can disrupt Qi flow thus augmenting any tendency to Stagnant Liver Qi. In Chinese medicine, the Liver is the general, the strategist responsible for the planning of life's activities and their timely occurrence.

THE PILL

Oral contraceptives have a two part mechanism. First they cause infertility by causing Liver Qi Stagnation. Then they promote menstruation by forcibly dredging the Liver. This leads to deeply entrenched Liver Qi aggravated by wasted or injured, Deficient Blood. Therefore, it is not surprising that the Pill is associated with the onset or aggravation of migraines in many women.

GLARE

The eyes are the orifice or opening of the Liver. Bright light is energy entering the system. Glaring, bright lights consume Liver Blood in the act of seeing them. This consumption of Liver Blood may tip the balance towards an Excess of Qi and Deficiency of Blood with the Qi venting upwards. It is also possible that the light may directly augment the Qi of the Liver. Unfortunately, exoteric

Chinese medicine does not discuss the influence of light and various colors on health and disease.

WEATHER

Chinese medicine emphasizes humanity's place in the larger, macrocosmic world. That place is pivotal, but still, we are part of that larger world, not it part of us. Therefore, what goes on inside of us is very much dependent on and reflective of what is going on outside. Any other point of view is sheer arrogance on humanity's part. In terms of migraines, different weather will aggravate different persons' migraines depending upon their individual Chinese diagnoses.

In Chinese medicine, wind is the meteorological Qi associated with the Liver. Generally, wind aggravates all Liver Excess conditions. Therefore, many peoples' migraines will be triggered by windy weather and especially hot, dry winds which are Yang on top of Yang. Persons aggravated by wind usually suffer from Liver Excess and Hot conditions.

Low pressure fronts are associated with damp, humid, overcast weather. This weather typically aggravates or initiates migraines in persons with Damp, weak Spleens. This Dampness further weakens the Spleen and hinders the free flow of Qi. This makes the Liver all that much more outrageous.

Cold weather and/or exposure to cold foods, such as ice-cream and frozen yogurt, can also precipitate migraines in some people. Cold has a tendency to constrict the flow of Qi and Blood. Cold weather causes constriction on the outside of the body causing increase of Heat and pressure within. Often this is enough to augment an already over-stuffed Chinese Liver.

HOT BATHS

Hot baths are dispersing and discharging. For some persons on the verge of a migraine, this dispersion and discharge causes venting upwards of pent-up Liver Qi. For other persons in whom the Qi has not accumulated to such a precarious point, a hot bath may actually abort an attack by bleeding off the Qi.

HYPERTENSION, TOOTHACHE, SINUSITIS, & TRIGEMINAL NEURALGIA

Most hypertension and trigeminal neuralgia are due to Excess Liver Yang and Heat ascending to the upper part of the body. Therefore, it is easy to understand their association with migraines. Also, many cases of sinusitis, especially chronic, recurrent sinusitis, are due to Liver Heat being transferred to the Gallbladder and thence to the sinuses via the Gallbladder Meridian. In such cases, an association with migraine is also easy to understand.

Toothache is usually of two types in Chinese medicine. One is Excess Stomach Fire and the other is Deficient Kidney Yin giving rise to Upward Flaring of Deficiency Fire. Stomach Fire may give rise to or aggravate Liver Fire. Whereas, Kidney Yin Deficiency may allow Arrogant Ascension of Liver Yang. Therefore, some tendency for toothaches of either kind to be associated with migraine is not theoretically out of line according to Chinese disease mechanism logic.

HEAD COLDS & HAYFEVER

Often, so-called head colds are a combination of Wind Heat mixed with or mutually aggravating Liver Heat. In such cases, it is the Liver Heat which gives rise to a simultaneous migraine, not the Wind Heat per se. Also, upper respiratory allergies in many Americans are due to rebellious Qi and Liver Heat stemming from Stagnation. The runny noses are due to this upwardly ascending Liver Qi and Heat drafting with it Dampness from the Spleen. This upward drafting may escalate into a more violent venting, in which case migraine may occur.

EPILEPSY, STROKE, & MIGRAINE

All three, epilepsy, stroke, and migraine are very similar in their disease mechanism according to Chinese medical theory. The main difference is their severity, not their mechanism. In other words, they are different quantitatively but not qualitatively. In all three cases, pent-up Qi from the Liver explodes or thrusts upwards through the core to the head where its further dispersion and discharge are hampered by the bony box which is the cranium.

As a hierarchy, stroke is the worst case scenario; epilepsy is the middle most; and migraines are the least serious of the three conditions. However, as we have seen, in certain instances, migraines can include many of the characteristics of stroke and seizures, such as convulsions, tremor, paralysis, paresthesia, and loss of consciousness. All are species of Wind disease, remembering that Internal Wind is nothing other than rebellious, erratic, violent Qi. Stroke and epilepsy usually also are complicated by some element of Phlegm; whereas, migraine often is not.

Although stroke, epilepsy, and migraine are obviously not all the same, single named disease (unless that name is apoplexy), they are, nevertheless, three stages of a single continuum. Apoplexy comes from the Greek *apo* or away from and *plessein*, to strike. The person with apoplexy has been stricken by an up-rushing energy within and that energy is pent-up, Stagnant Qi from the Liver.

THE RELATIONSHIP BETWEEN TENSION HEADACHES & MIGRAINE

Tension headaches are also due to an up-flushing of energy and usually from the Liver. However, the Qi which accumulates in the musculature of the neck and head is usually released much more slowly than the Qi which rushes up to cause migraine. In the case of tension headache, this up-flushing, rebellious, or errant Qi finds its way into the *Jing Jin* or Tendinomuscular Channels which are a relatively superficial level of Qi flow. This congestion causes muscular tightness and pain, including trigger points. Most often, this tightness and pain follow the pathways and spill-over areas associated with the Gallbladder Tendinomuscular Meridian. Because these *Jing Jin* do connect with each other, the Tendinomuscular Meridians associated with the Stomach and Bladder may also be effected.

In both the case of tension headache and migraine, it is Yang Qi flushing up causing the pain. In the first case, the Qi flushes up slowly and continuously into relatively superficial areas. In the second, the Qi flushes up abruptly and relatively more deeply. It does not have the time to dissipate towards the Surface. However, it is easy to see how one could experience a mixed headache which begins as a tension headache and becomes a migraine or vice versa.

CHINESE PREVENTIVE REGIMES

There are three basic preventive regimes which every migraine sufferer should consider carefully. These are deep relaxation, exercise, and diet. The first two are a Yin Yang pair. As mentioned above, most migraines have a component of pent-up Liver Qi. This is like pressure in a pressure cooker. When a pressure cooker comes to pressure, there are two ways that pressure can be relieved. One is to turn off or turn down the heat, and the other is to open the release valve. Migraines are the body's blowing the release valve as a last resort with the Liver Qi venting upwards as Wind and Fire through the core of the body to the head. However, we can turn down the heat by developing our ability to relax, and we can open the release valve before it blows by regular aerobic exercise.

DEEP RELAXATION

When Qi becomes pent-up, all that needs to happen to restore internal harmony is to allow that Qi to flow without impediment again. In this way, it will dissipate itself naturally and without incident. Our daily life here in the mechanized, modern West is inherently stressful beyond the healthy carrying capacity of the human organism. Although most of us can only make relatively small changes in the world around us, we can, however, change how we react to the world. Our response to stress is more important than the source of the stress itself, and our responses are largely a product of unconscious habit. Habit is established by repetition, and the best thing about bad habits is that they can be supplanted, granted if only slowly and perseveringly, by good habits.

Through daily, persevering, and deliberate practice, we can reprogram our bodyminds to react to stress in a relaxed and somewhat carefree way, rather than the tense, tight holding patterns most of us rely on. Daily, programmed deep relaxation is, I believe, the single most important element in disease prevention in young and middle-aged, urban and suburban American adults. For deep relaxation to be therapeutically effective, it must fulfill four criteria.

First, it must be done daily. The prescription I give my patients is every day for the first one hundred days without missing a single day. Then, in the next one thousand days, if one misses a few days, that's no problem. Without routine, day in, day out practice, although each individual session will feel refreshing, there will not be marked progressive and cumulative benefit. Therefore, deep relaxation needs to become a non-discretionary part of every day, as vitally important as eating and sleeping.

Secondly, each day's deep relaxation should last at least twenty continuous minutes. More than thirty minutes and there is no further health gain for that session. Less than twenty minutes and one will not get any appreciable health result. Therefore, we can say there is a twenty minute threshold to effective, therapeutic deep relaxation.

Third, the deep relaxation should result in complete somatic or physical relaxation and not just mental equipoise. One's whole body, inside and out, should become relaxed, soft, pliable, and at ease. All one's muscles, beginning from the head and working down to the feet, should be allowed to relax, expand, become heavy and warm. Then, in addition, one should calm one's mind through the use of an affirmation, such as the word "relax".

And fourth, having relaxed every muscle in the body, one should center their consciousness in their lower abdomen. One should breath in and out from their lower abdomen and experience their sense of self from that spot.

If one follows such a regime for one hundred days, their circulation and body temperature will improve, their digestion, elimination, and appetite will improve, and their sleep, mood, and energy will all also improve. Since these are the key criteria for good health in Chinese medicine, one can readily appreciate how important such deep relaxation is in maintaining good health in our hectic world.

Such deep relaxation is not the same as sleep. It is important not to fall asleep until after the twenty minute threshold is reached. After that, it is fine if one chooses to nap for a while or to go to sleep for the evening. Personally, I have found guided deep relaxation tapes, available at most healthfood and New Age bookstores, to be the easiest and most efficient way of fulfilling this deep relaxation prescription. One simply turns on the tape, lies down, and follows the spoken directions.

After having established the habit of complete and total relaxation, when one is out in the world and problems occur, as soon as one recognizes the tension building in their body, one simply lets go and relaxes. The longer one practices daily deep relaxation, the quicker one is able to let go and clear this tension. According to Chinese medicine, tension is impeded Qi and Blood and leads to both Heat and Stagnation. Therefore, the quicker we can let go and relax such tension, the less likely it is that pathologic Heat and Stagnation accumulate within us.

AEROBIC EXERCISE

Chinese medicine believes that a certain amount of physical exercise is necessary to maintain one's health and to prevent disease. Exercise speeds up a sluggish metabolism and, therefore, increases production of Qi and Blood. Deficiency of Qi and Blood can be due just as much to too little exercise as to over-exercise and exhaustion. In addition, regular physical exercise also helps sweep away and disperse any of the Six Stagnations discussed above. Exercise can, as it were, blow out the tubes Stagnant Qi, Blood, Food, Damp, Phlegm, and Fire. Since these are the main obstructing factors in most chronic, internal disease, one can readily appreciate the healthful and preventive benefits of regular exercise.

As with deep relaxation, I usually write my patients a "prescription" for exercise. For young and middle-aged patients I suggest some sort of aerobic exercise. Any activity which raises the pulse 85% above its resting level and keeps it there for a continuous twenty minutes is aerobic. And, just as with deep relaxation, there is a twenty minute threshold. If one exercises aerobically for from twenty to thirty minutes every other day, one will experience progressively better health. Again, one's circulation and body temperature will improve as will one's digestion, elimination, and appetite. One's mood and energy will improve and so will one's sleep.

In Chinese medicine, we believe that the Liver is the primary Organ effected by and involved in Stagnant Qi. Chinese medicine says the Liver stores the Blood. When we rest or are physically inactive, the Blood returns to the Liver from the periphery. When we exercise or are physically active, the Qi mobilizes the Blood out of the Liver. This mobilization helps to sweep away with it any Stagnant Qi or Blood. Also, aerobic exercise benefits the Heart and Lungs. The Lungs, in particular, are said to control the Liver according to *Ke* cycle energetics. Regular aerobic exercise can keep the Lungs strong so that the Liver is kept under control. In Chinese medicine, it is the Lungs that propel the Qi while it is the Liver which maintains its free flow and patency. In terms of migraine specifically, it is also believed that the Liver is responsible for sending up and the Lungs for sending down. Therefore it is obvious that the Liver and the Lungs have a close, reciprocal relationship vis a vis the Qi. Patients have consistently reported to me that regular exercise greatly reduces the severity of any symptoms associated with Stagnant Qi and Blood.

As mentioned above, stress, aka Stagnant Qi, is like steam in a pressure cooker. We can relieve this pressure by either opening the release valve or turning down the heat. Aerobic exercise is equivalent to opening the release valve within the body. It blows off the steam of accumulated Qi due to tension and stress. Deep relaxation is like turning down the heat under the pot. When regular aerobic exercise is coordinated with daily deep relaxation, one has a most effective and efficient combination for preventing stress-induced disease. The key to both is regularity and perseverance. Deep relaxation should be done every day and aerobic exercise every other day or not less than every seventy-two hours.

DIET

Chinese medicine places great importance on diet. We manufacture Qi and Blood to power and nourish us from a combination of three basic sources. The air we breath is mixed or "combusted" with the food and liquids we eat and drink catalyzed by our innate constitutional or inherent energy. There is little we can do about the air we breath and breathing is best left as an unconscious activity. Likewise, our constitutional or inherent energy is what it is and is not subject to much conscious modification by us. But what we eat, how much we eat, and how we eat are all within our control and can greatly effect our health and well-being.

To understand Chinese dietary theory, one must understand the Chinese concept of digestion. Everything that is eaten and drunk is first received by the Stomach. The Stomach is likened to a pot on a stove. Its job is to cook the digestate similar to a sour mash. As the digestate is "cooked" by the Stomach, it is "rottened and ripened". The Pure Essence of the digestate is then distilled by the Spleen and sent up to the Lungs and Heart to be transformed into Qi and Blood respectively. Therefore, before any nutritive essence can be absorbed by the body, the food eaten must be turned into 100 degree soup in the Stomach.

This explains Chinese medicine's emphasis on cooked as opposed to raw foods. Cooking is predigesting. By cooking, we begin on the outside of the body the process of rottening and ripening the Stomach must continue on the inside. Cooking makes the nutrients in foods more easily assimilable. Since the process of digestion is characterized as a process of Warm transformation, eating cooked, Warm foods results in a greater net gain. As the Pure arises to be transformed into Qi and Blood, the Turbid residue of the digestate is descended to be eventually excreted from the body. If the Pure and Turbid do not separate completely and efficiently, Dampness,

Phlegm, and Stagnant Food are created which obstruct the flow of Qi and the creation of Blood and generally gum up the works.

Likewise, since life is Qi and Qi is Warm, most food we eat should not only be warm in temperature but also Warm in nature. Chinese medicine identifies the inherent temperature of each food's Qi. Food can either be Hot, Warm, Neutral, Cool, or Cold. Mostly our diet should be composed of Warm and Neutral foods. And naturally, most foods are Warm or Neutral in temperature. However, many fruits and some vegetables, such as cucumbers, celery, and lettuce, are Cool or Cold. For a description of the temperatures of one hundred fifty commonly eaten foods, the interested reader is referred to my and Honora Lee Wolfe's *Prince Wen Hui's Cook: Chinese Dietary Therapy*.[92]

In addition, drinking too much liquid and especially cold liquids with meals dilutes the soup and smothers the Fire of digestion. A teacup of warm, boiled water, tea, or broth aids digestion, but an eight ounce glass of iced water or soda puts the Fire of digestion out temporarily. Therefore, in Asia it is traditionally believed that for optimal digestion the Stomach should be half full of food, one quarter full of liquid, and one quarter empty to allow for proper churning of the digestate.

There are also certain specific foods which should be eaten in great moderation by everyone and especially by anyone prone to migraines, whether classical, common, or cluster. Sugar is extremely Sweet. The Sweet flavor, according to Chinese medicine, goes right to the Spleen and also promotes the secretion of Body Fluids. Sugar is so Sweet that it "blows out" the Spleen. Rather than tonifying or strengthening the Spleen as does the natural, low concentrated Sweet flavor of most grains, meats, and vegetables, concentrated Sweet weakens the Spleen and therefore the healthy creation of Qi and Blood. In addition, sugar and other concentrated sweets such as honey, molasses, maple syrup, and various malt syrups, also tend to create Dampness due to over-secretion of Body Fluids. This Dampness then hinders Spleen function even more. The *Nei Jing*, the oldest classic of Chinese medicine, says that the Sweet flavor helps to relax the Liver and so it is natural for people with Liver Qi Congestion to crave the Sweet flavor. Unfortunately, when this craving is indulged by eating something so extremely Sweet as sugar, although it may give temporary respite, it only makes the entire situation that much more complicated and difficult to remedy. Placing a drop of Stevia tincture on the tongue when the craving for sweets arises can help alleviate this draving without causing the same reactions as sweets and sugar.

Other foods that can create Dampness are nuts, oils, and fats, chocolate, beef and pork, dairy products, eggs, and citrus fruits, pineapples, apples, and pears. Those whose Spleens are chronically Damp due to long-term Spleen Deficiency in turn aggravated by Liver Qi should be very careful not to over-eat Damp-producing foods. Alcohol is Dampening and also Hot. Therefore, it tends to create not only Dampness but Damp Heat.

Most spices are Hot in nature or, at best, Warm. In small amounts they, therefore, aid digestions, but, if over-eaten, they tend to create Excess Heat in the Stomach and Liver. Most Americans with migraine headaches or any disorder with a component of Liver Qi must be careful of Hot, Spicy foods. Spices and Pungent foods do decongest Stagnant Qi temporarily, but they also tend to waste the Blood and over-heat a typically over-heated system. Alcohol likewise temporarily disperses Stagnant Qi, but it too aggravates any pathologic Heat.

One other food which is a disaster for anyone with any Chinese Liver condition is coffee. This includes both caffeinated coffee and de-caff. Coffee disperses Stagnant Qi but wastes the Blood and Yin. As a Qi decongestant, it is extremely effective short-term as is alcohol to an alcoholic. Coffee gives a sense of energy and get up and go by freeing up stuck Qi. But in the process, it also liberates stored *Jing* or Essence in the Kidneys and, therefore, is deleterious to the health over-all. Although caffeinated coffee has an even worse effect than de-caff, it is not the caffeine alone that is the offending substance. There are many volatile oils in the coffee bean which as a whole cause the problem. Relatively speaking, green tea has caffeine but does not cause the same problems as even de-caffeinated coffee. In fact, green tea has many positive health benefits. Coffee, like sugar and alcohol is an addictive substance and is not easy to relinquish. Placing a drop of White Flower Oil on the tip of the tongue when the coffee craving strikes can help alleviate this dependency.

Professional practitioners of Chinese medicine can help design both remedial and preventive dietary treatment plans based on an individual person's Chinese diagnosis. Depending upon on that diagnosis, certain specific foods are more provocative and unbalancing than others. By basing dietary therapy on such a professional diagnosis, it is likely that one's diet will be more liberal than if one simply avoids everything that has caused anyone's migraines. For instance, persons suffering from a Damp and Deficient Spleen can often eat more Hot, Spicy foods than those whose diagnosis is Liver/Stomach Fire Blazing Upwards. The first person needs to be particularly careful about Cold foods, Damp foods, and excess liquid consumption with meals. The second person actually should eat more Cold and raw food to cool their Excess Heat.

When diet is an integral part of a multimodal treatment plan, the goal is that the migraine sufferer should be able to resume eating a moderate amount of the presently provocative foods once their system has been brought back to relative balance. That takes time, as in months and years, but in three to five years, if their total treatment plan has been effective, they should be able to enjoy small to moderate amounts of almost anything without provoking a migrainous attack. On the other hand, because each of us has an innate constitutional imbalance or predisposition, that does not mean we will ever be able to freely indulge and over-eat certain extreme foods. Most of the foods implicated as stimuli of migraines are energetically extreme and should not be eaten all that often by anyone.

This all means that persons living in a temperate climate should eat mostly cooked grains and vegetables. They should probably eat small amounts of meat, once every other day or so. By small amounts, I mean not more than two ounces per serving. Also, meat broths are very nutritious without the heaviness and Dampness of eating the flesh itself. Soups are very healthy since they already are extremely digestible. One can also eat occasional fruits, some nuts, and some dairy if one's digestion and elimination are sound and if they are not prone to Phlegm and Dampness. This is similar to the Pritikin diet or the Macrobiotic diet except without the emphasis on exotic Japanese foods often encountered in the latter. This is the diet most humans have eaten in temperate climates for thousands, if not tens of thousands of years. When looked at through the lens of history, our modern American diet is a recent fad of not much more than fifty years duration. By returning our emphasis to cooked grains and cooked, fresh vegetables, we fuel ourselves on the diet our bodies evolved on.

This is also basically the diet recommended in the National Research Council's *Diet and Health: Implications for Reducing Chronic Disease Risk*. According to this recently released, 1,300 page document, fats should make up no more than 30% of the total day's calories and saturated fats should only make up a third of that. Complex carbohydrates which are found in vegetables, legumes, and grains should make up at least 55% of daily calories. Protein for adults should *not* exceed any more than twice the daily recommended allowance (0.8 grams per kilogram of ideal body weight). Also according to this report, alcohol should be limited to one ounce per day and salt to a maximum of approximately one teaspoon per day.[93] Chinese medicine has been counselling such moderation in diet for well over a thousand years.

These three therapies described above -- deep relaxation, aerobic exercise, and dietary therapy -- are the three cornerstones of both preventing the arisal of disease and of treating chronic disease. Sun Si-miao, the most famous Chinese physician of the Tang dynasty (circa 700 CE), said that disease should first be treated by diet and lifestyle modification. If that does not cure the problem, only then should acupuncture and herbal medicine be employed. Sun Si-miao was writing in a simpler time and modern patients both want and probably need more professional intervention at the same time as they change their diet and lifestyle. Still, Sun's advice concerning the primary importance of these three, free therapies remains true to this day. Lucy Mall, writing in *Vegetarian Times*, states:

> Conventional medicine has ignored prevention

> until very recently, and the results are clear. Chronic illness is now responsible for more than 80 percent of all deaths and an even higher percentage of all total disability, states Robert A. Anderson, M.D., in *Wellness Medicine*. Many studies confirm that lifestyle factors, which are largely preventable, are the cause of debilitating disorders. In a Massachusetts study, for example, four risk factors for chronic disease -- lack of exercise, smoking, overweight, and alcohol use -- may account for over half the annual deaths in the United States, the authors concluded.[94]

In my experience, as much as seventy-five percent of all overt symptomology can be relieved in the majority of cases after three months of the above three, self-administered therapies. It is very common for me to meet patients on the street whom I have not seen for some time. Often they tell me that when their signs and symptoms flare up or return, all they have to do is get these three free therapies back on line again and soon their condition returns to normal. Sometimes they tell me this almost apologetically, as if my feelings will be hurt because they do not need my professional assistance. However, just the contrary, this is what causes me the greatest delight. The same Sun Si-miao also said the Superior Physician does not just treat disease but teaches society and helps form the intentions of humanity.

These free therapies -- deep relaxation, aerobic exercise, and dietary modification and moderation -- are the keys to preventing migraine headaches in the majority of migraine sufferers. They are also the first and most important parts in the treatment of migraines by full-spectrum, holistic, Chinese medicine. If persons afflicted by classical, common, and cluster migraines adjust their diets and lifestyles according to the above guidelines, then Chinese herbal medicine and acupuncture can bring the benefits of Chinese medicine into full display.

MASSAGE THERAPY

Massage therapy is one of the best and most enjoyable preventive therapies there is. Massage therapy is capable of releasing pent-up tension and, therefore, Stagnant Qi and Blood. It helps to transport and transform accumulated Fluids and Phlegm and combines the benefits of both exercise and deep relaxation. And it feels good to get.

Regularly scheduled, full-body massage can help reduce the frequency and severity of migraines in those whose migraines are due, in part, to stress. In order for massage to be prophylactic, it is best received once per week or not less than once every two weeks. Typically, a full-body, stress-reduction, and general, health-enhancing massage lasts from one to one and a half hours.

For those who tend towards Yin Deficiency with hyperactivity of Yang, oil medium massage is best. Massage with oil is especially effective for reducing and calming errant Qi flushing upwards and to the Surface in Yin Deficient, Flaring Fire persons. However, oil may aggravate those who tend to be Damp and Phlegmatic. These persons should receive a non-medium massage, such as Shiatsu performed on the clothed body, or a powder medium massage performed directly on the skin. Finely ground flour made of mung beans is good for those who are Phlegmatic and Hot. Rice flour is good as a massage powder for those who are Phlegmatic and Damp.

Regular massage can help teach a person how to relax. Having had a deeply soothing and relaxing massage, a person has a better idea of what they are aiming at feeling when they do their daily deep relaxation therapy. Stress reduction is cumulative. The more one relaxes, the more one can relax, and there is very little as relaxing as a full-body massage.

Unfortunately, all too few Americans are aware of the healing benefits of massage. Most Americans have never received a professional, non-sexual, therapeutic massage. And amongst those Americans "into" alternative therapies, massage is all too often over-looked because of its seeming lack of technological sophistication. However, as a preventive and health-maintenance therapy, massage is extremely effective. Therapeutic massage should be an integral part of a comprehensive Chinese medical healthcare plan. There are medical massage clinics in almost every traditional Chinese medical hospital in China, and traditionally, massage therapists could be found in every barber shop, public bath, hotel, and on many street corners throughout Asia. Although most Westerners equate Chinese medicine with acupuncture and Chinese herbs, massage is a definite and not to be forgotten part of traditional Chinese medicine.

CHINESE FIRST AID FOR MIGRAINES

Traditional Chinese medicine has a number of self-administered, first aid therapies for the immediate relief of migraine headaches. Some of these are ancient Chinese folk remedies and others are based on the professional logic of Chinese medicine. Not everyone of the following first aid remedies will relieve every individual's migraine. However, within this group of remedies, most migraineurs will find individual remedies which will work for them.

The first and one of the most effective first aid remedies for migraine is inhalation therapy. This is the breathing in through the nose smoke produced from the burning of medicinal substances. One Chinese folk remedy is to mix equal parts of borneol and camphor in a ceramic bowl and light this mixture with a match. The aromatic fumes from these medicinals will ignite readily. After allowing the mixture to burn briefly, one blows out the flame and then inhales the white smoke which arises. Usually one inhales this smoke between six and a dozen times. This can be repeated several times at intervals as needed. These two substances can be obtained from professional practitioners of Chinese medicine. They are quite inexpensive and have a long shelf life if kept in a tightly sealed container.

In Tibet, currently a province of China, various inhalant formulas are made for the treatment of migraines from a variety of herbs. Most of these formulas contain as their major ingredient, however, Lignum Aquilariae Agallochae or Eaglewood. This is a very precious, aromatic wood which has a profound effect on the energy or Qi. In Chinese medicine, Aquilaria is one of the most subtle of the Qi-regulating medicinals. One famous Tibetan inhalant prescription is called Agar 31, *agar* being the Sanskrit-Tibetan name for Aquilaria. This formula contains altogether 31 ingredients. It is sold in the United States as a stick incense called Nirvana marketed by the Himalayan Herb Co. This company's address is P.O. Box 8, Gangtok, Sikkim, India, and it can be ordered directly through the mail from India. It is also sold in this country in bookstores specializing in Tibetan and Buddhist books.

Where this complex formula is unavailable, one can simply burn powdered aquilaria on an incense charcoal and inhale the smoke from this a dozen or so times at intervals as needed. Lignum Aquilaria Agallochae can also be obtained from professional practitioners of Chinese medicine and at Chinese apothecaries in Chinatowns throughout the United States.

A third inhalant therapy is very effective and does not require any medicinal ingredients to perform. At any given time, we each are breathing primarily out of one nostril at a time. Usually the breath switches from one nostril to the other every forty-five minutes or so. According to ancient Oriental theory, our nostrils are connected to various Channels within the body, and, by deliberately choosing which nostril we are breathing through, we can alter our bodymind's metabolism and mood. When one feels a migraine coming on, one should immediately check which nostril one is primarily breathing through. Then one should close that nostril and breathe through the opposite nostril for sometime. This method is effective for aborting one-sided migraines if done at the very first premonition of an attack.

The fourth and final inhalant therapy also requires no medicinal substances. As one experiences a migraine coming on, one makes a conscious and deliberate attempt to do deep, abdominal breathing. One visualizes a spot one hand-span below the navel and one third of the way into the abdomen. Then one tries to feel and visualize the breath coming down to this spot with each inhalation. As one inhales, one expands their lower abdomen, and as one exhales, one contracts their lower abdomen. This is a version of a very ancient and widely practiced Oriental yogic technique which centers the Qi in the vital Root of energy in the Lower Burner. It has many health and longevity-promoting benefits beyond relieving migraines and can be practiced by anyone as a daily health-enhancing regime.

In Asia, the Qi, breath, and the mind are all almost identical. Therefore, it is logical that working with the breath is the most direct way of working with the Qi. Migraine headaches are more often than not a manifestation of upwardly perverting Qi. Because of that, inhalation therapy is one of the most immediate ways we can regulate this counterflow Qi. Internally ingested medicines must be digested and go through the Stomach before they begin to work, but the breath and inhaled medicinals carried by the breath go directly to work on the Qi. It is also possible to combine deep abdominal breathing with one nostril breathing and an herbal inhalant for even more effective first aid relief.

Because most migraines are upwardly rebelling Qi which has come apart from its Root in the lower abdomen, there are a number of ways to pull this Qi back down and out of the head. Although we talk about Liver Qi, Spleen Qi, Kidney Qi, etc., all the Qi of the body is connected and of a piece. Therefore, anything which pulls Qi to the lower half of the body may be useful for lessening or aborting a migraine headache. The following methods can be selected from based on individual experience, preference, and availability. All are based on the logic of Chinese medicine vis a vis the Qi.

For persons who are basically Hot and Excess, treading in ankle deep cold water in a bathtub is one method of pulling Qi back down in the body. The Qi is mobilized to the feet to warm the cold being experienced in that part of the body. This then subtracts from the total volume of Qi thrusting upwards into the head. A variation of this is plunging one's hands into cold or ice water. Individuals who are Cold and Deficient should only use these methods with care, as they may further weaken an over-burdened Spleen and allow the Liver to become all the more Excess. Since both Excess Hot and Deficient Cold persons may have chronically cold hands and feet, it is best to allow a professional practitioner of Chinese medicine make this determination.

Another variation on this technique is to put ice or cold packs on the bottom of the feet and hot packs on the head or base of the neck. The cold packs tend to draw some of the Qi downwards; while the hot packs open the Channels and Collaterals in the head to allow the Qi and Blood more unobstructed space to flow through. The hot packs decrease the pain; while the simultaneous cold packs seek to abort the violent uprising.

One can also do something very similar by acupressure. Acupressure is the pressing of acupuncture points for first aid relief. In order to open the Channels and Collaterals in the head, one can massage the base of the skull and the fleshy webs between the thumbs and forefingers with as much pressure as one can bear. One can also massage between the big and first toes and the space behind and to the side of the ball of the feet with a pincher movement of the fingers and thumbs. This helps draw arrogantly ascending Liver Qi back down to the lower half of the body. Either of these two methods can be combined with hot or cold packs if only one of these is available. In which case, one combines one opening method for the head and one downward leading method for the feet.

Another method of leading Qi down in the body is to eat. This is especially effective if the migraine is preceded by intense hunger. Eating centers the Qi in the midsection or Middle Burner of the body and draws it out of the upper half. This method will not work if the person is already nauseous but can be effective if resorted to before the attack has gone that far.

Likewise, sex can sometimes abort an incipient migraine by first drawing the Qi and Yang to the genitals and then dispersing it to the Surface with orgasm. Although some peoples' migraines are triggered by sex, others' can be aborted by sex. This includes masturbation. Again, this will only work to a marked degree at the first sign of a headache. Once the headache has established itself, most people cannot conceive of sex. We are all familiar with the line, "Honey, not tonight; I have a headache."

Persons whose migrainous attacks are associated with constipation can immediately try taking an enema. Enemas are the quickest and most immediate way of purging Heat from the Liver via the

Intestines. Because of the close connection between the Liver, Intestines, and the Lungs, an enema can disperse Stagnant Liver Qi and regulate downward upwardly rebellious Qi. Purgatives do the same thing but are mostly too slow to stop a migraine which has already begun.

For those who experience nausea, chills, and vomiting as part of their migraines, there is a very effective Chinese herbal decoction that usually can abort or alleviate this particular type of migraine within fifteen to twenty minutes. The formula is called Wu Zhu Yu Tang (Evodia Decoction) in Chinese. Although it takes twenty minutes to prepare, its effect is so predictably good when migraine is accompanied by nausea, chills, and a vomitaceous feeling that it is recommended that anyone suffering from this type of migraine keep this medicine on hand. It can be purchased from professional practitioners of Chinese medicine or at Chinese apothecaries. These herbs will keep for three years without problem if kept in an air-tight, dark container. Be sure to tell the apothecary or practitioner to adjust the standard formula to be more effective for headache. This is done by adding four or five more ingredients which specifically de-obstruct the various Channels of the head.

The final self-administered first aid treatment for migraines which have already begun is to drink strong tea or coffee. Chinese doctors usually suggest tea since it disperses Excess Qi and Internal Heat. However, coffee will also do this. In Chinese medicine, there is a famous first aid herbal remedy for headache called Chuan Xiong Cha Tiao San (Cnidium & Tea Regulating Powder). This prescription is drunk with strong tea. It is available in pill form from Chinese medical practitioners or again at Chinese apothecaries. For first aid use, these pills should be chewed in the mouth before swallowing; their effect will be quicker. Also, one can take double or even triple the recommended dose on the package without fear of over-dosing. This prescription is effective no matter where the pain is felt on the head since it includes ingredients which de-obstruct all the Channels of the head. Migraineurs should always keep a supply of these pills on hand. However, if these pills are not available, strong tea or coffee alone can be used.

CHINESE REMEDIAL TREATMENT FOR MIGRAINES

CHINESE HERBAL MEDICINE

Chinese medicine's main professional therapy is internally administered herbal medicine. Actually, herbal medicine is a bit of a misnomer. Although most of the 5,000 medicinal substances in Chinese medicine come from various plants, Chinese medicine does also use both naturally occurring mineral substances and animal by-products. All these ingredients are seldom used singly. Most often they are combined into formulas comprised of from eight to fifteen ingredients. In such a formula, the ingredients work synergistically. Some of the ingredients boost each other's beneficial, therapeutic effect. Other ingredients are meant to negate possible side-effects. And yet other ingredients insure that the right effect is obtained in the right part of the body.

The most common traditional method of administration is as a decoction. This means the herbs are boiled in water for forty-five minutes to an hour or more. After straining off the liquid, this "tea" is drunk several times per day. Other methods of administration include pills, powders, liquid and dried extracts, and syrups. Which method of administration is used will depend on the individual patient's diagnosis and case. However, commonly, one begins treatment with strong decoctions. As their symptoms improve and progress is made, they are then moved to powders, pills, or extracts for easier, long-term administration.

The practitioner of traditional Chinese medicine composes a customized herbal prescription specifically for the individual patient. He or she begins with the diagnosis of the disease category and the individual patient's Pattern of Disharmony. He or she then modifies the formula for the patient's idiosyncratic signs and symptoms and individual constitution. Therefore, a dozen patients all with a Western diagnosis of migraine may each receive a different herbal formula. For anyone whose migraine is periodic with the phases of the moon or for women with menstrual migraines, their formulas are adjusted approximately once per week depending upon where the patient is in their cycle, what symptoms are currently manifesting, the season of the year, the phase of the moon, the weather, and any of a number of other individualized considerations.

When prescribed correctly based on an individualized Chinese energetic diagnosis, Chinese herbal medicine is free from *any* side-effects. Since Chinese medicine sees the organism as a whole, throwing one part of the body out of balance in an attempt to heal another part makes little sense. Chinese doctors are constantly updating and modifying their patients' treatment since the patient is constantly changing in relationship to their environment.

Therefore, it is very important for the patient to keep their Chinese physician constantly informed about all their body functions and symptomatic experiences. Likewise, it is also important that the Chinese doctor monitor their patients' pulse and tongue on a regular basis since an accurate traditional Chinese medical diagnosis primarily depends upon the comparison of a patient's signs and symptoms, tongue, and pulse.

In my experience, the longer a person has suffered from migraines, the longer it takes to achieve significant results with Chinese medicine. Generally, I suggest one month of treatment for each year a person has suffered from migraines. Simple Excesses of short duration are relatively easier and quicker to treat. Whereas, Mixed Excess/Deficiencies or simple Deficiency conditions usually require longer treatment. If a disease condition has persisted for a long time, there is usually some element of Stagnant Blood in the *Luo Mai* or fine capillary beds which is difficult to remedy. However, persistence is what pays off in Chinese medicine. When looked at from day to day, a year or more seems like a long time, but when looked at in relation to how long a condition has persisted, significant amelioration in one year may not seem like such a bad deal in retrospect.

When treating migraine headaches, we generally do not expect any crises as part of the treatment plan. That means we do not try to initiate or provoke any acute discharges as do some other forms of natural healing. Rather, we expect a gradual improvement in the patient's condition with consistently less frequent and less severe headaches. At the outset, while the Chinese diagnosis and, therefore, the treatment are still just working hypotheses, there may be some ups and downs and some adjustments to be made. But typically, there are no or few crises in the Chinese treatment of migraines.

Some people may at first think that Chinese herbal medicine is expensive. It can cost, depending upon the method of administration, dose, and prescription, from one to four or even five dollars per day. However, when compared to the cost of most Western drugs and medical procedures, the net cost of Chinese medicine is relatively cheap. Why some Americans may hesitate or balk at spending this much money on Chinese herbs is that they feel Chinese medicine is just an experiment. Since they are not sure it will work for them, it seems an expensive risk. However, Chinese medicine is hardly experimental. It has been developed by over 100 generations of literate professional practitioners who traditionally were regarded as some of the most educated persons within their society. It is a logical, rational system of medicine, which has proven itself as consistently and emperically efficacious in clinical practice. When compared to the cost of most Western medicine, Chinese medicine is comparatively inexpensive.

Some people may also find the taste of Chinese herbal decoctions very bitter and unpleasant. In China there is a saying, the bitterer the brew, the better the medicine. However, that may be small consolation for the modern American patient. But, I can say based on my own and my patients' experience, when a Chinese herbal prescription matches exactly an individual patient's condition, after the first few doses, the body recognizes the benefit of the decoction and even comes to crave the taste of such bitter brews. When this happens, it is a very encouraging sign. Then, if and when the same formula begins to taste bad again, it is a sign that the current prescription is no longer exactly right and needs to be modified or changed completely to a different formula.

As the patient's situation improves, the professional practitioner is often able to switch the patient from a strong herbal decoction to an easier, ready-made prescription. This may be in the form of a powdered, desiccated extract, tablets, pills, or a tincture. This makes it easier for the patient to take their medicine over an extended period of time and is often also less expensive. Most often, patients are advised to take Chinese medicine for some time after the elimination of all their symptoms so as to consolidate the therapeutic effect and prevent a relapse. Many patients, after they finish their course of treatment, take periodic doses of Chinese medicine in order to prevent a recurrence based on seasonal cyclicity or when they are under particular stress. Usually, ready-made Chinese herbal medicines can be kept for from one to three years and retain their medicinal efficacy.

Chinese herbal medicine is a fine art which takes a great deal of education and years of practice to master. Chinese herbal ingredients are medicinals. They are medicine and are not just inconsequential dietary supplements. As such, they must be prescribed by professional practitioners specifically trained in Chinese herbalism and their prescription must be based on traditional Chinese theories and a traditional Chinese energetic diagnosis. Chinese doctors have developed and refined this system over two thousand years. When Westerners attempt to use Chinese medicinals on the basis of a Western diagnosis or Western medical theories alone, either the treatment is not successful or, in fact, iatrogenic complications are caused. Chinese medicine may be "herbal", but it is strong medicine none the less. When practiced and prescribed professionally and correctly, it is strongly beneficial.

ACUPUNCTURE

Acupuncture is the other main, professionally administered

therapy of traditional Chinese medicine. Acupuncture is the insertion of extremely fine needles into specific locations on the body called acupoints. According to Chinese medical theory, Qi and Blood flow through the body over discrete Channels and Vessels. These *Jing Mai* are relatively the same for everyone regardless of race. Located on these pathways are points or "switches" at which the energy travelling through them can be manipulated and therapeutically adjusted. Inserting needles into these points is similar to flicking switches or circuit breakers in an electrical system. The acupuncturist can either send more or less energy to an Organ or area of the body, can direct the Qi, Blood, and Body Fluids, can speed up or slow down these Humors, and can warm them up or cool them down.

The needles are inserted from just barely under the skin to a half inch, one inch, or even more in depth. Patients may experience the slightest pinch on insertion and then any of several sensations as the needle touches the point which is below the skin. These sensations can include tingling, heat, distention, heaviness, soreness, or an electrical, nervy feeling. These are all good signs that the needle has "tapped the Qi" and that something therapeutic is happening. Usually somwhere around eight points are needled in a single treatment (often bilaterally) and the needles may be left in place for from fifteen to twenty minutes as the patient lies on the table. If the acupoints have been correctly selected, typically patients will begin to breath very deeply. They will relax deeply and may even fall asleep. These are all good signs the treatment is restoring balance to the body and is freeing stuck and stagnated energy and tension.

Acupuncture can be used in two ways in the treatment of migraine headaches. First, it can be integrated in a comprehensive treatment plan attempting to get at the energetic root of the problem. When used in conjunction with Chinese herbal medicine, acupuncture is administered once per week. In a few cases, such as cluster headaches, where headaches are occurring several times per week or more, acupuncture may be done every day, every other day, or three times per week. However, once the cluster or series of headaches has abated, on-going treatment is usually once per week.

Acupuncture is the direct manipulation and balancing of the patient's Qi flow, and, because of that, it can have very profound effects on the bodymind. Acupuncture touches the Qi of the patient in a very subtle way, different from herbal therapy. It can free the Qi flow on the mental-emotional level in a much more direct way than can internal medicine. Of the two, acupuncture can catalyze the seemingly more magical and profound changes in a person's whole being and balance. Therefore, because most migraines are an expression of errant or rebellious Qi, I highly recommend regularly scheduled acupuncture treatment in conjunction with internal Chinese herbal medicine.

The second way which acupuncture can be used in a comprehensive treatment plan for migraines is for professional first aid relief of headaches in progress. Through insertion of needles in acupoints adjacent to the areas of pain, the acupuncturist can immediately destagnate the congested Qi and Blood, thus relieving the pressure. Then, through needling acupoints on the arms and legs, he or she can also reroute the rebellious up-rising Qi so that it does not jam and cram into the head.

Acupuncture can typically begin to relieve the pain of migraines within moments of insertion of the needles, and patients can feel the pressure in their heads disperse and become more diffuse moment by moment. Many times, patients have been literally carried into my office sunk in their pain and misery and yet recovering and being communicative again within minutes of needling. In a few cases, acupuncture temporarily intensifies and accelerates the pain, bringing the attack much more quickly to a crescendo and resolving crisis ending in vomiting or diarrhea. But most often, acupuncture immediately and unequivocally reduces the pain and shortens the course of acute migrainous attacks, including cluster headaches.

When acupuncture is used for first aid pain relief, the points are somewhat different from those used preventively during regularly scheduled, weekly appointments. During the acute phase, more attention is placed on local points on the head and empirical points for control of associated symptoms, such as nausea and vomiting. Whereas, during regularly scheduled visits between headaches, emphasis is placed on deep harmonization of the Qi, Blood, and Internal Organs in an attempt to rectify the problem at its root.

The following is a review of the research on the value of acupuncture in the treatment of migraine. In general, it is quite positive and my experience is that these improval or amelioration rates can themselves be improved when acupuncture treatments are individually tailored to individuals' Chinese diagnoses and when acupuncture is only one part of a comprehensive traditional Chinese treatment plan.

Form 1976 to 1978, the Ludwig-Boltzmann Institute for Acupuncture in Vienna studied the effects of acupuncture on 68 migraineurs. They reported that of these 68, 2/3 got good to very results, 1/8 moderate results, and 1/4 no results at all.[95] Another study of 20 migraineurs conducted at the Postgraduate Institute of Medical Education and Research in Chandigarh, India reported that 30% of their patients experienced marked improvement, 35% improved by seventy-five percent, 25% got mild improvement, and 10% remained unimproved. This was based on each person receiving the same standard treatment over a course of ten treatments.[96] A third study conducted at the Salo District Health Care Center in Finland treated 115 migraineurs with a standardized course of treatment and individual follow-up treatments. 81% of these migraine sufferers experienced a mean reduction in their pain which lasted up to 56 months after the cessation of treatment. Further, only 5 out the 115 participants in this study did not get any relief and had to be maintained on their current Western drugs.[97]

A study conducted by the Department of Physiology at the University of Otago Medical School in New Zealand reported that of their 16 patients with migraine, 40% experienced a 50-100% reduction with less severe attacks and less nausea and vomiting.[98] Whereas, a study conducted in the People's Republic of China (where, it is presumed, the level of acupuncture proficiency should be quite high) reported a 93.5% effectiveness in 31 patients who had all failed to respond to Western medicine. This was utilizing a standard treatment repeated every other day.[99] Likewise, a study of 48 migraineurs conducted at the National hospital for Nervous

Diseases in London reported that 24 out of 41 patients treated (56%) improved with acupuncture compared to 9 of 36 responding to Western medicine.[100]

Looking at the above statistics and considering that, with the exception of the Chinese study, none of the practitioners were professionally trained Chinese doctors but were rather Western MDs and medical researchers, I think it is safe to say that more than 50% of migraine sufferers can be helped by acupuncture.

Sometimes, acupuncturists attempting to treat migraine headaches must also withdraw Stagnant Blood from the system. This may be done by tapping the superficial *Luo Mai* or Collaterals with a small hammer with tiny needles embedded in its head. This causes just a little bit of bleeding over the area tapped which, in turn, discharges Stagnant Blood and activates the flow of fresh Blood through these Collaterals or capillaries. In other cases, the acupuncturist may prick engorged and purple veins and capillaries found on areas of the body, like the torso and legs, distal to the head. Only a very small amount of typically dark, lifeless, Stagnant Blood is bled from these veins and the treatment is no more painful than pricking one's thumb with a rose briar. Often such bleeding of the Collaterals and the direct expulsion of Stagnant Blood is the sine qua non of successfully treating chronic, long-term migrainous pain. When such superficial veins are bled, contemporary practitioners use sterile bleeding lancets identical to those used by MDs.

Here in the United States, most practitioners of traditional Chinese medicine are also trained acupuncturists. There is a National Commission for the Certification of Acupuncturists which offers a national board certification exam. Acupuncturists who are nationally board certified typically append Dipl. Ac. for Diplomate of Acupuncture after their names. Just as one would not hire a plumber to do electrical wiring, patients should best receive acupuncture from trained, credentialed, professional acupuncturists. Also, because of the advent of AIDS, most American acupuncturists use ethylene oxide gas sterilized, disposable needles. This virtually eliminates *any* possibility of cross infection through contaminated needles. In addition, more and more insurance companies are willing to reimburse for acupuncture since it is such a cost-effective therapy.

DURATION OF TREATMENT & COMPLIANCE

Traditional Chinese medicine is a natural medicine, an Oriental naturopathy. In general, it uses safe and non-toxic treatments with no or low iatrogenic impact in an effort to re-establish balance within the patient and between the patient and their larger environment. The practitioner of Chinese medicine seeks to nudge the body's own homeostatic mechanisms just enough for the body to right itself. Chinese medicine does not try to force changes on the bodymind but rather provides the opportunity, the space for the bodymind to itself instinctively move towards greater health and ease.

Because the professional practitioner of traditional Chinese medicine works in concord with nature and not against it, Chinese medicine, like most natural medicines, works slower and more smoothly than modern Western medicine. Therefore, the prospective patient must be willing to give Chinese medicine a chance to do its job at the body's own pace. As mentioned above, one month of healing for each year a chronic condition has persisted is a generous and realistic time-frame. At first, this may look like the "never never" plan. But, when viewed from the perspective of a seventy year plus life span, six months, a year, a year and a half, or even two is actually a short time *if* real, deep health and balance are obtained.

Having practiced traditional Chinese medicine here in the United States for more than ten years, it is clear that those patients who stick with Chinese medicine for more than sixth months get the best and most profound results. In Chinese medicine, traditionally, a doctor could not claim a cure until the patient was able to go through all four seasons without a relapse or recurrence. The sweetest music to my ears is when patients tell me two or three years after having undergone a course of Chinese medical treatment how consistently better and better they feel once having been pointed in the right direction.

Unfortunately, we live in such a hurry-up world that many contemporary patients find it difficult to persevere in a single therapy for more than a few weeks or, at most, a couple of months. There are so many options in the healthcare marketplace, and it is difficult not to want to do them all, all at once. "If a little is good, more must be better." But not in Chinese medicine.

Professional Chinese medicine is based on the Doctrine of the Mean, the way of moderation. When seeking balance, more than enough of anything will tip the balance, and once that balance has been tipped, the bodymind will tend to swing erratically for some time. Therefore, it is important to discuss with the professional practitioner of Chinese medicine any therapeutic input from other sources. Chinese medicine has the theoretical breadth of vision to potentially describe any input into a person's system, whether that input or stimulus was known in ancient China or not. The professional practitioner can help the patient decide what foods, vitamins and minerals, and over the counter medicines are appropriate based on their individualized Chinese energetic diagnosis. In general, symptomatic shotgun therapy is best avoided. It rarely results in actual balance.

The treatment plan of deep relaxation, aerobic exercise, diet, herbal medicine, and acupuncture outlined above is a comprehensive and holistic treatment plan which seeks not only to allay symptoms but also to restore balance at a deep level of one's being. In my experience, the better the patient's compliance and the more persevering their following of the total treatment plan, the better the therapeutic result. Following such a comprehensive treatment plan takes some determination. It is not without its difficulties. But, not only will one's migraines show marked improvement, the patient's entire health and well-being will take a turn for the better. As in the story of the turtle and the hare, it is slow and steady which wins this race. It is little wonder that the turtle is a traditional Chinese symbol of longevity.

FINDING A PRACTITIONER OF TRADITIONAL CHINESE MEDICINE

Traditional Chinese medicine is a rapidly rising star within the American alternative healthcare community. As of this writing, there are more than twenty American schools and colleges of acupuncture and Chinese medicine. That means that the number of professional American practitioners of this art is growing by about five hundred practitioners per year. Many American practitioners have also either gone to medical school in Asia or have gone to Asia for post-graduate training. And, of course, many Asian doctors have immigrated to the United States in the last twenty years.

In addition, there is a National Council of Acupuncture Schools and Colleges which helps to over-see and regulate the quality of training and education, a National Commission for the Certification of Acupuncturists which helps to insure minimum, entry level, professional competence, and various state and national professional associations, such as the American Association of Acupuncture and Oriental Medicine, which help to regulate professional ethics, network amongst practitioners, and provide continuing, post-graduate education. Acupuncture has now been legalized as a state-approved healthcare modality in over a score of states and in many others, favorable legislation is in the process of being enacted.

In states where acupuncture is licensed and state regulated, one should be able to find the names of local practitioners in the yellow pages of their phone book or by contacting their state Department of Health, Board of Medical Examiners, or Department of

Regulatory Agencies. In such states, it is wise to insure that potential practitioners are, in fact, state licensed. In states without licensure, it is best to seek out those practitioners who are nationally board certified. Such practitioners typically append the initials Dipl. Ac., for Diplomate of Acupuncture, after their names. These national board exams insure minimal professional competency and not less than the equivalent of two full years of academic and clinical training specifically in acupuncture.

In the United States, not all acupuncturists are practitioners of Chinese herbal medicine, but almost without exception, all American practitioners of Chinese herbal medicine are also acupuncturists. As yet, only a handful of states include Chinese herbal education and examination in their licensing and, until now, there is no national herbal board exam. Therefore, it is important to query potential practitioners on the school, nature, and extent of their Chinese herbal training. In general, the practice of Chinese internal or herbal medicine is more demanding and requires more education and experience than the practice of acupuncture. Hopefully, in the near future, there will be some kind of national credentialing of traditional Chinese herbalists.

When searching out a qualified and knowledgeable practitioner, satisfied, word of mouth referrals are important. Therefore, it is also appropriate to ask for references from previous patients treated for the same problem. Likewise, it is important that the practitioner be able to communicate with the patient in order to explain their Chinese diagnosis and the rationale behind their treatment plan. In all cases, a professional practitioner of Chinese medicine should be able and willing to give a written traditional Chinese diagnosis of the patient's case. Also, I personally suggest that patients select practitioners who belong to both local and national Chinese medicine/acupuncture professional associations. Such associations offer referrals of professional members in good standing and high repute. In addition, such associations almost always have a code of professional ethics which their members promise to uphold and this further insures the quality and professionalism of the care they provide.

Traditional Chinese medicine, including acupuncture, is a discrete and independent healthcare profession. It is not a technique to be added to the bag of tricks of some other profession. It takes just as long *or longer* to learn Chinese medicine and acupuncture as it does to learn allopathy, chiropractic, naturopathy, or homeopathy, and previous training in one of these systems in no way confers *a priori* competence or knowledge in Chinese medicine or acupuncture. Therefore, I heartily advise prospective patients seeking to avail themselves of the benefits of traditional Chinese medicine to seek out professionally trained practitioners of this system. As suggested above, just as one would not hire a plumber to do electrical wiring, so patients should receive Chinese medicine from professionally trained practitioners of Chinese medicine.

For further information regarding the American practice of Chinese medicine and acupuncture and for referrals to local professional associations and practitioners, prospective patients may contact:

National Acupuncture Headquarters
Washington, D.C.
(202) 265-2287

This is the joint offices of the American Association of Acupuncture and Oriental Medicine, the National Commission for the Certification of Acupuncturists, and the National Council of Acupuncture Schools and Colleges.

CONCLUSION

The purpose of writing this book has been to share with Americans the knowledge that traditional Chinese medicine can effectively and cost-efficiently treat and cure neurovascular headaches. It is my hope that if more Westerners knew about the effectiveness of traditional Chinese medicine in treating such headaches, more migraine sufferers would seek out and begin Chinese style treatment as a *first option* early on when their condition is still relatively simple and easy to remedy. This could save a great deal of both physical and emotional pain for American migraineurs who are already under such great personal and societal stress.

Secondly, if more Americans experienced the effectiveness of traditional Chinese medicine in dealing with these specific conditions. These same persons would be all the more likely to seek traditional Chinese healthcare for other illnesses and complaints as would their friends and relatives. This would then help to popularize the use of traditional Chinese medicine in this country which, I believe, would be a great boon for the health of this nation.

And third, it has been my intention in writing this book to share with my countrymen and women the rational and holistic vision of Chinese medicine. Traditional Chinese medicine is not just a collection of exotic and outlandish, empirical therapies. Rather, its greatest treasure is its humane and rational explanation of why and how we as humans living in this world get sick the way we do. Chinese medicine offers us the opportunity to take responsibility for and to regain control over our own health and well-being.

Ultimately, it is a blueprint for living a healthy, sane, and harmonious life.

APPENDIX I

An Historical Review & Comparison of Western & Chinese Medicine Vis a Vis Migraines

Some Westerners reading this book on the traditional Chinese medical treatment of migraines may feel that Chinese medicine is an exotic import and, as such, is irrelevant to our experience as Americans. Although Chinese medicine historically was founded in China, as a system of medicine, it transcends cultural and ethnic limitations. If Chinese medicine is valuable in the late 20th century West, it is because it is the clearest surviving, mature, and clinically professional version of the traditional medicine which was once universally found around the world.

Most traditional healing systems share common concepts of humoral and vitalist theory. Humoral theory describes basic substances in the body which, when they vary in relative proportions, account for many of the various fluctuations in health and well-being. Vitalist theory posits the existence of a vital force which animates the bodymind, as it does all of nature, and which flows through the body over discreet pathways. Although the details of humoral theory and vitalism may differ from culture to culture, age to age, yet there is a remarkable consistency to these theories once one penetrates superficial semantic differences. This consistency suggests a common felt reality experiencable by all people at all times.

When one compares the Chinese description of the disease mechanism at the root of most migraines with Western medical theories before the mid-19th century, one is struck by the essential identity of these descriptions. Professional medicine in the West from the time of Hippocrates and Galen two thousand years ago through the Renaissance and into the Age of Reason is known as Scholastic medicine, the medicine taught in the *schola* of the monasteries during the Middle Ages and at the universities during the Renaissance. This Scholastic medicine was developed from the works of such Greek and Roman physicians as Hippocrates of Cos and Galen of Rome. After the fall of Rome, it was adopted and further refined by the great Arab physicians, such as Ibn Sena (Avicenna) and Al Rhazes. These Arab doctors combined Greco-Roman medicine with Chinese and Ayurvedic medicine which flowed West over the Silk Road and then transmitted this back to the Europeans during the Crusades and the Christian reconquest of Spain.

As a practitioner of traditional Chinese medicine, I am very comfortable with the Scholastic humoral and vitalist descriptions of migraine dating from before the 1850's. They are in no fundamental way different from traditional Chinese descriptions. According to Scholastic medicine, migraines are most often due to an excess of yellow or black bile. It was such excesses of the choleric or melancholic humors which were believed to be associated with feeling *liverish*, of being in a *black humor*, or of having a *jaundiced* point of view. Such excesses were also associated with *bilious* vomiting and the gastric upset of a "sick-headache". Although humoralists obviously emphasized the humors, it is easy to see the identity between Liver Qi Stagnation/Depression and an excess of Yellow or Black Bile. And just as the Chinese physician cures by re-establishing healthy balance, the Scholastic humoralist had exactly the same therapeutic intention. As Alexander Trallianus stated:

> If therefore headache frequently arises on account of a superfluity of bilious humor, the cure of it must be affected by means of remedies which purge and draw away the bilious humor.[101]

Contemporaneous with such humoralist theories were vitalist theories sometimes referred to as "sympathetic". According to sympathetic concepts of the flow of vital energy over pathways linking distant parts of the body, "migraine has a peripheral origin in one or more of the viscera (the stomach, the bowel, the uterus, etc.), from which it is propagated about the body by a special form of internal, visceral communication; this occult form of communication, hidden from and below the transactions of consciousness, was termed 'sympathy' by the Greeks, and 'consensus' by the Romans, and was conceived to be of particular importance in connecting the head to the viscera (*mirum inter caput et viscera commercium*)."[102] The practitioner of Chinese medicine has no trouble visualizing these pathways connecting the head with the Stomach, Uterus, Large Intestine, and the Liver. These are the Channels and Collaterals of Chinese acupuncture theory, and the vital force which communicates over these and makes these "suffer together" (sympathy) is the Chinese Qi and Blood. When one recognizes the Bile as the humoral expression of Liver Qi and adds to this the interconnectedness of the Liver, Stomach, Large Intestine, Uterus, and the head, one has essentially the same picture of upwardly perverse Liver Qi venting into the head of traditional Chinese medicine. Alexander Trallianus' "superfluity of bilious humor" mentioned above not only means an excess of bilious humor but that it flows (*fluidus* from *fluere*, to flow) up (*super* meaning literally above). This description was pragmatically accurate enough so that Thomas Willis, a physician writing in the late 1600s was still comfortable describing pathways linking the uterus and the head and thus explaining menstrual migraines and the tendency of more women than men to experience migraines.[103]

Acceptance of the traditional Chinese medical theories on the cause and treatment of migraine headaches is, therefore, not the acceptance of some foreign and outlandish doctrine. Rather, it is a return to the ancient, clinically applicable and humanely pragmatic wisdom which is the common root of most traditional medical systems worldwide. Western Scholastic medicine is, for all intents and purposes here in the West, a dead medicine. Although it survives as Islamic Unani medicine in India, Pakistan, Afghanistan, and Iran, its lineage in the West has lapsed irreparably. The living lineage of traditional Chinese medicine, on the other hand, has never lapsed in more than two thousand years. As a medical system, it is remarkably alive and well and even flourishing worldwide. It has held its own as an equally useful, valuable, and professional medicine alongside modern Western medicine in China, Korea, Japan, Taiwan, Hong Kong, Vietnam, and Singapore and has been endorsed for worldwide propagation by the United Nations.

Modern Western medicine is founded upon philosophical materialism and its most reactionary proponents take pride in their rejection of vitalism. But vitalism, the belief in a living spirit animating all of reality, is central to the living, human experience. Modern Western medicine has made some very wonderful discoveries and is very useful in certain situations. But the contemporary healthcare consumer does not have the faith he or she once had in this flashy yet myopic system.

The limitations of Western medicine are the same as its greatest ability, the ability to focus in seeming isolation on very small bits of information. Leaving aside for the moment the epistemological fallacy that anything can be studied in isolation, in this process of reductionism, modern Western medicine has lost sight of the big picture. In the struggle to reintegrate this larger, living, and holistic vision back into professional medicine, Chinese medicine is destined to be a major factor in the development of a New Medicine for the 21st century. Ironically, this is only the latest swing of a perennial pendulum back towards the humoral and vitalist visions which have always been the basis of medicine in the West up until the fairly recent past.

APPENDIX II

Traditional Chinese Descriptions of The Use & Abuse of the Most Commonly Prescribed Western Medicines for Migraine

This book's main purpose is to introduce to the American public the benefits of traditional Chinese medicine for the prevention and treatment of migraines. However, although Chinese herbal medicine and acupuncture are specifically Chinese therapies which can be effectively employed in a comprehensive and holistic treatment plan for migraines, the most important part of Chinese medicine is its ability to describe the phenomenal world vis a vis health and disease in a more wise, humane, and empowering way. Traditional Chinese medicine's description of the disease mechanisms of migraine make sense on a felt human level, and, based on these descriptions, patients themselves can understand how they can prevent and control their migraines through lifestyle modifications, dietary therapy, and various self-employed regimes. But Chinese medical theory is broad enough and universal enough to also describe other therapies and medicines not specifically Chinese and to incorporate them, where beneficial, into its panoply of cures.

Traditional Chinese medical theory can describe, for instance, the medicinal properties and actions of Western pharmaceuticals as if they were traditional Chinese "herbal" medicines, remembering that Chinese medicine has always used medicinals from all three kingdoms, animal, vegetable, and mineral. By describing the properties and actions of modern pharmaceuticals according to traditional Chinese terminology and methodology, we can gain the same human-level wisdom about these as about more traditionally Chinese medicinals, such as Ginseng and Dang Gui. With this information, we can make a wiser and more discriminating use of these pharmaceuticals. We can make use of all the speed and specificity of modern pharmaceuticals and avoid or mitigate their often deleterious side-effects. Causing side-effects means causing imbalances in the total organism. This is like stealing from Peter to pay Paul. Chinese medicine considers this unacceptable except in a few, short-term cases. However, by employing these methods sparingly and on a selected basis in turn based on the theories and 2000 plus year experience of Chinese medicine, we can make use of these powerful medicines. In short, traditional Chinese medical theory is so wise and universally valid that it can encompass all of modern Western medicine so that we can, to some extent, have our cake and eat it too.

The main Western pharmaceuticals used in the treatment of migraines today are propranolol, clonidine, ergotamine, diazepam, phenobarbital, methysergide, caffeine, and aspirin. Some of these are prescribed preventively and others are administered for relief of a headache in progress. The names given above are the generic names. However, each of these in the United States also has one or more proprietary names, which, in fact, are generally the more familiar.

PROPRANOLOL

Propranolol is more commonly known as Inderal and Inderide. It is a Beta-blocking, anti-hypertensive medication which is used in the treatment of angina pectoris, high blood pressure, heart arrhythmias, and migraine headaches. In the case of migraines, it is prescribed preventively to reduce the frequency and severity of migraines. It is not a first aid medication.

When attempting to describe a new medicinal according to the terminology and methodology of Chinese medicine, we must analyze both the drug's intended symptomatic use and its side-effects. Then we look for the common Chinese mechanisms which allow us to understand why the drug can alleviate certain symptoms and yet causes others. What we are looking for is a common denominator, the line of action in Chinese medicine which ties together all symptomatic information about the medicinal. Therefore, besides its indications, what are Inderal's contraindications and side-effects?

First of all, persons with asthma and hayfever should not take Inderal. Its expected or "natural" side-effects are lethargy, fatiguability, cold hands and feet, and orthostatic hypotension, i.e. dizziness upon standing. Its mild adverse reactions are skin rashes, temporary loss of hair, drug-induced fever, reduced appetite, nausea, vomiting, diarrhea, insomnia, and vivid dreaming. Inderal's serious adverse reactions include disorientation, confusion, hallucinations, amnesia, emotional depression, and increased risk of asthma. Moderate over-dose results in general weakness, slow pulse, and orthostatic hypotension. Large over-dose causes fainting, a weak and slow pulse, cold, sweaty skin, and convulsions. In addition, one should not do isometric exercise while on Inderal and its use should not be discontinued abruptly.[104]

When indications, contraindications, and side-effects for Inderal are all taken into account, it becomes clear in terms of traditional Chinese medicine that this medicine is a "heavy" sedative. Heavy sedative in Chinese medical terminology does not just mean a strong sedative. It has a more technical, mechanical meaning as well. Heavy sedatives in Chinese medicine push down forcefully upwardly rebellious Yang. They are believed to literally weigh down, smother, and drag down up-rising Qi. Ascension of Liver Yang can cause angina, high blood pressure, arrhythmia, and migraine. Therefore, it is obvious why, from a Chinese point of view, Inderal treats all these particular conditions.

However, heavy sedatives depress the Clear Yang and ultimately harm both the Stomach/Spleen and the Qi. All the contraindications and side-effects of Inderal are either due to 1) this heavy sedation compressing already Stagnant Qi, as in asthma, depression, and skin rash; or 2) this heavy sedation causing Deficiency Injury of the Stomach/Spleen and Qi, such as the lethargy, fatigue, orthostatic hypotension, nausea, vomiting, etc. The fact that isometric exercise while on Inderal can cause a rise in blood pressure is due to the fact that Inderal itself compresses the Qi as it pushes it down from above. Isometrics cause further compression with inevitable rise in internal pressure. As for sudden discontinuation, if Inderal is suddenly withdrawn, this compacted Qi held forcibly down may have a likely tendency to spring back upwards violently if the Qi has not become Deficient due to long-term use.

In terms of Inderal's safe usage based on traditional Chinese medical wisdom, it is all right to use Inderal to lower Arrogant Ascension of Liver Yang as long as there is also not a lot of Stagnant Liver Qi in the Middle and only for as long as the patient's Stomach/Spleen remain unharmed. Nausea, vomiting, and diarrhea are not considered acceptable side-effects in Chinese medicine since the Stomach/Spleen is the Root of Postnatal Qi and Blood production. Therefore, patients with weak or inharmonious Chinese Stomach/Spleen function should be screened against before being prescribed Inderal. This the professional practitioner of Chinese medicine can do based on tongue and pulse signs and symptoms ascertained through questioning.

CLONIDINE

Clonidine is sold in the United States under the names Catapres, Combipresen, and Dixarit. It too is an anti-hypertensive. Its side-effects are quite similar to Inderal's. For "natural", expected side-effects, Dr. James Long, M.D., lists drowsiness, dryness of the mouth and nose, constipation, and light-headedness upon arising. Its mild adverse effects are skin rash, hives, localized swellings, and itching; dizziness, depression, insomnia, and nightmares; nausea and vomiting; and dryness and burning of the eyes and breast enlargement. No serious side-effects are noted, but moderate over-dose results in marked drowsiness, weakness, and a slowed pulse; while a large over-dose causes deep sleep and lowered body temperature. Long-term use of clonidine can cause water retention and edema. It can also cause temporary sexual impotence, painful blanching and numbness of the hands and feet on exposure to cold, and may also aggravate the hypertensive response to isometric exercise also noted with Inderal.[105]

Clonidine, based on the above information, should also be categorized in Chinese medicine as a heavy sedative, one which forcibly lowers Yang energy. However, its harmful effects extend not only to the Stomach/Spleen but also to the Kidneys, the Root of Yang. This explains its causing sexual impotence and more painfully cold hands and feet. In particular, clonidine seems to have a pronounced adverse effect on Water metabolism, causing signs and symptoms of non-arisal of Fluids above and Water

Swelling or edema below. And finally, the fact that clonidine tends to cause depression, breast distention, constipation, and burning eyes in addition to just dryness suggests that it causes aggravation of Liver Qi, transforming it into Depressive Fire.

Therefore, clonidine also is probably not a good choice of treatment over any extended period of time. Especially it should be contraindicated in persons with weak Stomach/Spleen function and even more particularly in patients with poor transportation and transformation of Liquids. In addition, it should be used only with great care in persons with marked Liver Qi or Depressive Liver Fire and should not be used by persons with Kidney Yang Deficiency. For instance, many menopausal women with migraines have a combination of Arrogant Liver Yang with Liver Blood and Kidney Yin Deficiency *and* Kidney Yang Deficiency. These women should not take clonidine.

When any of such "heavy" Yang-depressing sedatives are used, their side-effects might be mitigated by combining them with the Chinese herbal ingredients in Chai Hu Long Gu Mu Li Tang (Bupleurum, Dragon Bone, & Oyster Shell Decoction) without the dragon bone and oyster shell which are themselves less powerful heavy sedatives. The other ingredients in this formula dating from the late Han dynasty, or almost 2000 years ago, are formulated to specifically deal with the exact kind of side-effects Inderal, clonidine, and other heavy sedatives tend to cause.

ERGOTAMINE

Ergotamine is marketed in America under the brand names Ergomar, Ergostat, Bellergal, Cafergot, Wigraine, etc. Dr. Sacks says that it is rarely used any more, but many of my migraine patients in Colorado have used it within the recent past. When it is used to treat migraine, it is only effective when taken immediately at the onset of the first signs and symptoms *before* the headache is established. Unfortunately, the typical necessary effective dose is often just short of a poisonous over-dose. Ergotamine is a very dangerous drug. It is primarily prescribed as a migraine analgesic but is sometimes also prescribed as a preventative.

Ergotamine's "natural" side-effects are cold hands and feet, mild numbness, and tingling. Its mild side-effects are localized swelling and itching; nausea, vomiting, and diarrhea; chest and muscle pain; headache, dizziness, confusion, and drowsiness. Its serious adverse reactions include gangrene of the intestine and extremities.[106]

According to Chinese medicine, ergotamine should be classified as a *Zhi Xue* or hemostatic medicinal. It stops the flow of Blood, and therefore Qi, by astringing or constricting the *Jing Mai* or Channels and Vessels. Such restriction of flow clamps down on the up-flushing Qi and Blood. However, this will only work if not too much Qi and Blood are already venting upward. Because Stomach/Spleen function depends upon the unrestricted flow of Qi up and down, ergotamine causes disharmony of the Middle Burner. In addition, all its other adverse signs and symptoms are due to its basically stopping the flow of Qi and Blood.

As a first aid measure, this may be all right in some cases. But it is a potentially dangerous approach and one which should only be resorted to occasionally. Chinese medicine deems the free flow of Qi and Blood to be of paramount importance in maintaining health and well-being. Most migraines are, in fact, due to retarded or constrained Qi and Blood flow. Ergotamine seeks to reassert restraint of pent-up Qi when that Qi has started to flow upwards out of control. Preventively, the patient usually needs to do just the opposite -- to maximize Qi flow so that there is no pathological accumulation.

DIAZEPAM

Diazepam is much more commonly known as Valium in the United States. It is one of the most frequently prescribed drugs in the Western world. Western MDs dispense Valium as a mild anti-anxiety tranquilizer. Its "natural", expected, and "unavoidable" drug reactions are drowsiness, lethargy, and unsteadiness in stance and gait. Its unusual, mild side-effects are skin rashes, dizziness, fainting, blurred vision, double vision, slurred speech, nausea, and menstrual irregularity. Valium's serious side-effects include jaundice, fever and sore throat, and, paradoxically, acute excitement, hallucinations, and rage. Other side-effects may include eye pain, glaucoma, and depression. Moderate over-dose results in marked drowsiness, weakness, a drunken feeling, staggering gait, and tremor. While large over-dose results in stupor progressing to deep sleep or coma.[107]

Valium is yet another heavy sedative according to Chinese medical theory. It forcefully restrains and suppresses ascendant Yang. However, based on the above drug reactions, I would say that Valium enters the Chinese Liver more than the Heart. Therefore, in Chinese medicine, one could say it *An Hun* or pacifies the Psyche associated with the Liver rather than *An Shen* or pacifies the Spirit in the Heart. Valium's paradoxical reactions are due to increased compression in the Liver due to its weighty lowering of Liver Yang. If there is imploded Liver Qi transforming into Depressive Liver Fire, such weighty compression only aggravates the transformation into pathologic Heat which then can, and, in some cases must explode to vent itself, as in acute excitement or rage. Therefore, Valium is not a very wise choice of medications for those persons suffering from Depressive Liver Qi unless it is administered with other medicinals which simultaneously dredge and relax the Liver and benefit the Stomach/Spleen.

PHENOBARBITAL

Phenobarbital or phenobarbitone is dispensed in the United States as Barbita, Luminal, Sedadrops, Solfoton, Solu-barb, and numerous other brand names. It is a mild, sleep-inducing barbiturate used at low dosages to relieve mild to moderate anxiety, at higher dosages to induce sleep, and continuously to prevent epileptiform seizures.

Phenobarbital's "natural", expected, unavoidable side-effects include drowsiness, lethargy, and a sense of mental and physical sluggishness. Its mild, unexpected side-effects are skin rashes of various kinds, hives, localized swellings of the eyelids, face, and/or lips; dizziness, unsteadiness; nausea, vomiting, and diarrhea; and joint and muscle pain, particularly in the neck, shoulder, and arms. Phenobarbital's more serious adverse reactions are hepatitis with jaundice and severe skin reactions. Its idiosyncratic or paradoxical reactions include excitement and delirium.[108]

Here again we are dealing with a heavy sedative in Chinese medical terminology. In this case, we can say that phenobarbital enters the Liver *and* Gallbladder since it causes hepatitis and jaundice and seems to obstruct the *Shao Yang* Channel (neck, shoulder, and arms) associated with the Gallbladder. Its side-effects from over-dose and prolonged use are generally similar to those of other heavy sedatives we have described and phenobarbital's Chinese contraindications are essentially the same. It is interesting to note that phenobarbital decreases the efficacy of those Western drugs which dredge the Liver and activate the Qi and Blood, such as coumarin family anti-coagulants, aspirin, oral contraceptives (second phase), and phenylbutazone.

METHYSERGIDE

Methysergide, more commonly known as Sansert, is used exclusively for the prevention of neurovascular headaches, such as migraines and cluster headaches. According to Dr. Sacks, it is not prescribed much anymore[109], but, for a period of time, it was regarded as a drug of choice in the treatment of chronic or recurrent migraine. Sansert's "natural", expected side-effects are weight gain and fluid retention. Its mild adverse reactions are skin rashes, facial flushing, and transient loss of scalp hair; heartburn, nausea, vomiting, and diarrhea; drowsiness, dizziness, unsteadiness, and transient muscle and joint pains. Its serious adverse effects are nightmares, hallucinations, and acute mental disturbance; cold, numb, painful hands and feet; leg cramps when walking and pain in the chest, abdomen, or back; fatigue and/or fever; and urinary disturbance. Moderate over-dose results in nausea, vomiting, abdominal pain, diarrhea, and incoordination. Long-term use may result in fibrosis or scar tissue forming within the chest and obstructing the lungs, heart, and blood vessels. Abrupt discontinuation may result in "rebound" headaches.[110]

Sansert is probably more of an astringent, blood-stopping or *Zhi Xue* medicinal than a heavy Yang-suppressor. Most of its signs and symptoms seem to be about the restriction of Qi and Blood flow. It seems to me it enters the Liver and Spleen in particular, restricting Liver Blood and Spleen Qi. Weight gain and fluid retention are due, therefore, to inability of the Spleen to transport and transform Fluids. Based on such a description, patients diagnosed as suffering from *Si Ni*, inverted Qi flow of the four extremities due to Liver/Spleen disharmony, should not use this medicine. Since many women with Liver Qi Stagnation have *Si Ni*, this medicine should be especially carefully considered with females.

CAFFEINE

Caffeine has been used for centuries in the form of coffee, tea, and cocoa. However, as a pharmaceutical, it is sold singly under such names as Nodoz and Cafecon. As an ingredient in compound drugs, it is often combined with aspirin or with ergotamine. One caffeine-ergotamine combination specifically formulated for migraines is Cafergot. In Western medicine, caffeine is prescribed to prevent or relieve at the onset vascular headaches and to relieve drowsiness and mental fatigue.

Caffeine's "natural" side-effects include nervousness, insomnia, and increased urination with the degree of these reactions being proportional to the amount of caffeine taken. Its mild adverse effects are headache, irritability, lightheadedness, a drunken feeling, impaired thinking; and nausea, heartburn, indigestion, and stomach irritation. Caffeine's serious side-effects include development of gastric ulcers. Tolerance to caffeine decreases with age. Moderate over-dose results in nervousness, restlessness, insomnia, tremor, sweating, tinnitus, spots before the eyes, heart palpitations, and diarrhea. Large over-dose results in excitement, rapid and irregular pulse, rapid breathing, delirium, hallucinations, and convulsions. Possible effects of long-term use include development of duodenal and peptic ulcers and aggravation and perpetuation of fibrocystic breast disease.[111]

Caffeine should probably be classified as a Surface-relieving medicinal in Chinese medicine. Surface relievers are dispersing. They catalyze the release of Qi which flushes to the Surface throwing open the pores or what are called in Chinese the *Qi Men*, Gates of Qi. In general, Surface relievers stimulate the circulation of Qi and Blood. Caffeine catalyzes the transformation of *Jing* or stored Essence into Qi. Since this *Jing* is what ultimately nourishes the *Shen* Spirit and keeps it calm, exhaustion of this *Jing* and loss of this Qi through dispersion leads to nervousness, insomnia, palpitations, tremor, and sweating. Since this *Jing* is stored in the Kidneys, this dispersion also leads to polyuria and tinnitus, both symptoms of Kidney Deficiency. Surface-relieving, dispersing medicinals have a tendency to exhaust or waste the Yin in general, and it is caffeine's exhausting of Stomach Yin which leads to heartburn, gastritis, indigestion, and ulcers.

When taken for the relief of migraines, caffeine promotes the dispersion of Yang Qi rushing up into the head. Instead, it causes some of this Qi to be dispersed outward to be liberated through the skin. However, caffeine should not be used by persons who are Stomach Yin Deficient, Blood Deficient, or Heart and/or Kidney Yin Deficient. Since some migraines are due to Arrogant Ascension of Liver Yang *due* to Kidney Yin Deficiency, careful discrimination should be made by professional practitioners of Chinese medicine. In persons with relatively robust Yin, caffeine may be an acceptable first aid remedy. Since the process of aging is the process of the consumption and exhaustion of the Yin, caffeine should be used with care in the elderly. Since it is also implicated in breast, and possibly cervical disease, female patients should be screened for a tendency to these.

ASPIRIN

Aspirin is, technically, acetylsalicylic acid. However, in the United States, aspirin is an official generic designation. Salicylic acid occurs naturally in willow bark, birch bark, and aspen bark and has been used as a pain-reliever in various traditional cultures for centuries if not millennia. In Western medicine, aspirin is used to stop pain and to reduce fever. Recently it has also been used to prevent repeat heart attacks.

Although aspirin is a relatively safe medicinal, it does have some side-effects and contraindications. As for "natural", unavoidable side-effects, aspirin may cause mild drowsiness in sensitive individuals. Its mild adverse, unexpected side-effects include skin rash, hives, nasal discharge resembling hayfever, and nasal polyps. In addition, aspirin may cause stomach irritation, heartburn, nausea, and vomiting. Its serious side-effects are asthma, unusual bruising, anemia, erosion of the stomach lining with internal bleeding, fatigue, weakness, fever, sore throat, hemorrhaging, and hepatitis with jaundice. Moderate over-dose typically causes stomach distress, nausea, vomiting, tinnitus, dizziness, impaired hearing, drowsiness, and sweating. Large over-dose results in stupor, warm, dry skin, fever, deep and rapid breathing, fast pulse, muscular twitching, delirium, hallucinations, and convulsions[112] Persons scheduled for surgery are advised to discontinue aspirin use one week prior so as to avoid excessive bleeding.

Aspirin is just the opposite in function to ergotamine according to Chinese medical theory. Rather than stopping bleeding, aspirin activates the Blood causing it to flow quicker and more freely. In Chinese medicine, it should be categorized as a *Huo Xue* or Blood-activating, destagnating drug. However, Blood activators can cause excessive Blood flow and are, in general, dispersing and exhausting in nature. This is why aspirin relieves pain but also causes bleeding and why it causes anemia and drowsiness. When aspirin itself causes fever, this is due to its wasting the Blood and, therefore Yin and/or to its dispersion of Qi resulting in Deficiency fever. Aspirin, like caffeine, and for somewhat similar reasons, also injures Stomach Yin, thus causing heartburn, indigestion, nausea, vomiting, etc. The difference between aspirin and caffeine is that aspirin disperses the Blood and caffeine disperses the Qi. That is why both are often taken together for the treatment of headache and why they often do help. They do disperse and ease the congestion of Qi and Blood caused by up-flushing into the head. However, aspirin, like all *Huo Xue* medicinals, should be used with care so as to prevent injury to the Blood and Yin. In Chinese medicine, such *Huo Xue* medicinals are often prescribed with *Bu Xue* or Blood-tonifying medicinals to protect from such iatrogenic injury.

Western drugs, because they are highly refined and very specific, are powerful. They can be powerfully good or powerfully bad depending upon how wisely they are used. In the New Medicine which must emerge in the 21st century, Western pharmaceuticals will be used in tandem with more rounded, slower acting, safer, and more buffered, naturally occurring medicinals, such as herbs. In general, it is both my opinion and experience that traditional Chinese medicine is better than Western synthetic pharmaceuticals for long-term or preventive treatment. However, Western drugs are a wise and intelligent choice in the management of acute conditions as long as they are prescribed based on a discriminating differential diagnosis. The first rule of Western medicine is, "First do no harm". Ironically, it is traditional Chinese medicine which can provide the rationale and conceptual framework for administering Western drugs more safely based on better differential diagnosis taking into account the individual as a whole.

APPENDIX III

The Psycho-spiritual Aspects of Migraine

Consciousness in Chinese is called *Shen Ming*. *Shen* means Spirit and *Ming* means brightness. The word *Ming* is related in Chinese to the Fire Element or Phase. Chinese medical philosophy divides all of phenomenal reality into Yin and Yang. Yang is associated with Heaven and Yin with Earth. But in the human body, Yang manifests as Fire and Earth as Water. Ancient Chinese physicians were extremely perceptive and accurate in understanding that the living human organism is primarily water animated by a myriad of essentially Warm transformations. It is warmth or Fire which animates our being and distinguishes between life and death. When we are alive, we are warm, and when we are dead, we are stone cold.

The Root of all Fire in the human body is the *Ming Men Zhi Huo*, the Fire of the Gate of Life. This is also known in Chinese medicine as *Zhen Yang*, True Yang, *Shen Yang*, Kidney Yang, and *Shen Huo*, Kidney Fire. As these names imply, this heat is rooted in the Chinese concept of the Kidneys which are also called the *Xian Tian Zhi Ben*, the Before Heaven Root. *Xian Tian* is a very profound concept, difficult to translate into English. In English language Chinese medical texts, this term is often translated as Prenatal. However, Primordial is perhaps more correct in English, or Noumenal as opposed to Phenomenal. In any case, the Root of all heat and warmth in the human organism is the Kidneys.

This *Ming Men Huo* provides the warmth for the Stomach/Spleen to initiate their process of digestion. Likewise, it energizes Liver/Gallbladder function and the Heart and Lungs. In addition, it helps keep Fluids and Blood in the body moving and transforming. however, on a psycho-spiritual level, this Fire of life located in the lower abdomen or Lower Burner undergoes various transformations as it moves upwards in the body. Although it begins as heat, it must transform into light. This then is the light of the Spirit, consciousness, *Shen Ming*.

In exoteric or secular Chinese medicine, this arisal and transformation is described primarily as an interchange between the Kidneys and Heart mediated by the Stomach/Spleen and Liver. The Kidneys represent Water and the Heart, Fire. But within Kidney Water there is Fire, *Ming Men* Fire or Kidney Yang, and by the time this Fire reaches the Heart, it must or should be transformed into light, not heat--the light of Enlightenment. Obviously, for most of us, this transformation is far from being as complete as it could be, and in clinical practice, most manic or excitory psycho-emotional disturbance is due to the presence of pathogenic Fire or Heat in the Heart/Pericardium.

However, in esoteric Chinese mysticism or yoga, the *Ming Men* Fire rooted in the Kidneys rises up the back along the spine to enter the head or Brain. This is essentially identical to the arising of the Kundalini described in East Indian yoga. As this heat travels up the spine, it undergoes transformations as it passes through the various chakras or energy plexes, ultimately to become the *Shen Ming* when it fills the Brain. This then shines forth from the eyes as their clarity and vivacity. According to this esoteric tradition, the *Ming Men* is physically located just above the perineum in the area of the uterus in women and the prostate in men. This area is also often referred to in yogic literature as the first or root chakra.

Although these two descriptions of the arisal of the Fire of Life and its transformation into *Shen Ming* or consciousness appear anatomically contradictory, both are used by Chinese doctors depending upon what aspect of this arisal and transformation they are attempting to describe or manipulate. To Chinese practitioners, who often in the Ming and Qing dynasties belonged to secret societies somewhat analogous to the Masons in the West, both these models are pragmatically useful and are not considered mutually exclusive. No matter which model we chose, life and consciousness are seen as a combustion of matter and a transformation of substance into energy catalyzed by heat and producing both more heat, but more importantly, light.

This basic transformation is sometimes referred to as the *San Bao* or Three Treasures. These are *Jing*, the essential substance or material basis of incarnation; the Qi or energy which both transforms this substance but also is created by this transformation; and *Shen* or Spirit which is transformed out of the accumulation of Qi. Qi has five basic functions according to Chinese medical theory. It transports or moves; it transforms; it restrains, holds, or consolidates; it defends; and it warms. Qi is living warmth, the warmth of human life and metabolism. Qi is also Yang as opposed to substance being Yin. And Yang Qi has an innate tendency to rise.

The circulatory system over or through which the Qi flows is called in Chinese the *Jing Luo* or Channels and Collaterals. There are 365 Collaterals and *all* of these transport the Qi upwards to the head. This upward flow to the head is accomplished on several different levels of energy flow, from very superficial to core pathways. If it were not for this focusing of Qi towards the upper part of the body resulting in its transformation into *Shen*, there would be no consciousness.

In fact, in Chinese medicine, unconsciousness is *always* associated with some blockage or failure of the Clear Yang or Qi arising. For instance, at night, the Qi is relatively exhausted or depleted and so it sinks into the core of the body to recoup and regenerate. During this retreat phase, there is little or no consciousness. If a person faints because of being weak, this is because there is not enough Qi to arise as consciousness. If one faints due to fright, this is because their Qi is scattered and so there is not enough of it to coalesce into consciousness. The Clear Yang can also be obstructed in its upward flow to the Heart/Brain by Dampness, Phlegm, or Stagnant Blood. Any of these can impede or cause loss of consciousness. And finally, so much Qi may arise that it causes ruptures in its circulatory system. The system, as it were, explodes. And the Qi, not held within its Pathways, i.e. not coalesced sufficiently, dissipates and cannot pull itself together into consciousness.

There is normal consciousness and super-consciousness. By super-consciousness, I mean the expanded awareness associated with *exalted* or mystical states of mind. From a Chinese medical point of view, such super-conscious states are the result of more than normal amounts of Qi or Clear Yang (*Qing Yang*) arising into the Heart/Brain. It seems that there are some inherent checks or

Gates (*Men*) within the human organism which allow only so much of this Yang Qi to flow upward in most of us most of the time. But, if enough Yang Qi is generated or collected, these Gate mechanisms are breached and more than normal Clear Yang flows upwards to be experienced as more than normal consciousness or *Shen Ming*.

Yogic practices, in general, seek to accumulate Yang Qi and then to focus and direct it upward. This can be done through breathing since the Qi and breath are closely associated. It can be done through celibacy and certain sexual yogas since the *Jing* or Essence (of which the semen in men and Blood in women is the physical manifestation) is the material basis of the Qi. It can be done through assuming certain physical postures which focus and coerce or lead the Qi upward. And it can be done through meditation since the Qi and *Yi* or mind are essentially the two sides of a single reality. Most spiritual disciplines employ several of these techniques simultaneously or in succession, and the basic pattern to what in China is called Inner Alchemy (*Nei Dan*) and most other spiritual transformational processes is first a deliberate accumulation of *Jing Qi* and then a focusing and elevation of this, thus facilitating its transformation into more than normal *Shen Ming*. Therefore, we can speak of three phases in or aspects of the development of super-conscious states: augmentation, transformation, and elevation, with elevation and transformation occurring somewhat simultaneously.

Another way one can experience super-conscious states is through the use of psychedelic, *psychotropic* drugs, such as marijuana, peyote, mescaline, psilocybin, and LSD. These drugs throw open the normal checking Gate mechanisms, thus allowing the Clear Yang to rush upwards as is its natural wont. This explains the fact that these drugs only remain present in one's system a very short period of time, yet the psychedelic experience may last eight or more hours. The "*high*" itself is powered by the person's own Clear Yang liberated from its storehouse in the Lower Burner at the base of the spine. However, when this energy is spent, the person "comes down" and is left feeling "burnt out". In fact, all of the signs and symptoms of psychedelic burnout are Kidney Qi/Kidney *Jing* Deficiency signs complicated by the flaring of

Deficiency Fire. It takes approximately 30 days for the average person's Kidney *Jing* to recoup after a marijuana high and one to three years to recoup after an LSD trip. This Root Essence Qi is both spent and replaced geometrically, not arithmetically, and, therefore, a second trip coming closely on the heels of a first is not so, so debilitating. At the same time, it is also not so "high" or so powerful, since the energy is not yet there for the same display.

In my opinion, there are only small differences in mechanism between super-conscious states/mystical experiences on the one hand and strokes, epilepsy, and migraines on the other. These differences do have very large consequences for the individual involved and the society of which they are a part. But as phenomena, they are closely linked. In all four conditions, there is an augmentation of Qi which moves upwards in an abrupt and unusual way. In the case of most migraines, strokes, and seizures, the Yang energy accumulates in the Liver. This can be due to stress congesting and, therefore, backing up the flow of Qi in the Liver. Or it can be due to weak Kidney Yin failing to root the Yang in the Lower Burner. In both cases, the Yang accumulates to a certain point and then erupts up through the core of the body passing over the Diaphragm and flushing up into the head often drafting with it Phlegm and Dampness.

In the case of mystical experiences, the energy may first accumulate in the Lower Burner, not in the Liver, as a consequence not of stress but of deliberate practices designed to augment the Kidney *Jing* and strengthen the *Ming Men*. Then it may arise upwards through somewhat different pathways than migraines, strokes, and seizures. However, I can only say *may* because, in fact, many mystics have simultaneous or alternating histories of migraines and/or seizures and mystical states. The visions of St, Hildegard of Bingen are now recognized as migrainous displays by Western doctors. But, are they *only* migraines?

As a clinician, I have personally treated individuals sometimes referred to as "Kundalini casualties". These are people who experience genuine mystical states of consciousness complicated by various related health problems, such as headaches and seizures. The Shakers and Quakers of American religious history

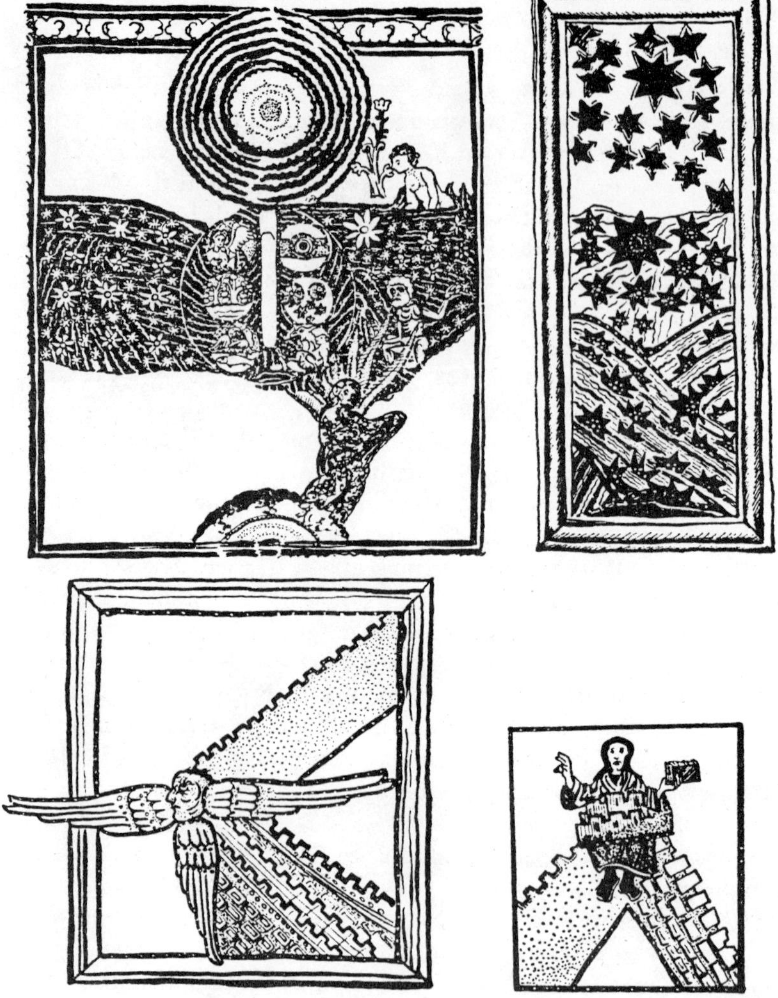

Figure 24. Varieties of migraine hallucination represented in the visions of Hildegard

and many Christian charismatics of today are also examples of the close relationship between seizures and convulsions and mystical, ecstatic experiences. As a yogin myself, I have likewise experienced seizures and convulsions interspersed with various altered states of consciousness when in retreat. And it is a common phenomenon that many religions either consciously or unconsciously create a great deal of emotional stress as part of their path.

The purpose of this discussion is not to reduce or devalue religious or mystical experiences. On the contrary, my purpose is to suggest to migraineurs that there is the possibility of apotheosis in their pain. What I mean is that, instead of regarding our migraines as a curse, we could understand them as a basically spiritual urge to perfection gone just slightly awry. They are a symptom both of our urge to perfection and the fact that we are not yet perfect on a relative level. As such, they are an undeniable call to action, one that is hard to forget or dismiss.

It is my opinion that the incidence of migraine is, in fact, increasing in our increasingly pressurized society. We are becoming both more secular and materialist *and* religious and spiritual at the same time. There is only one urge. But how we respond to that urge takes us either to heaven or hell. On an individual level, we either facilitate our arisal and transformation of Clear Yang or we eventually explode, as in stroke and heart attack. On a planetary level, we either evolve and transcend our basest motives or blow ourselves up altogether. This process is built into the very fabric of our being, but how we experience and relate to it is our choice.

Paradoxically, the various experiences we have in altered states of consciousness are themselves not the actual goal. The goal is to recognize that no experience, whether of heaven or hell, ever actually touches us -- that the nature of mind is not affected by the contents or experiences of the mind. However, because of the intensity of altered states of consciousness, and because during such states our normal habitual conceptual patterns are interrupted, it is more likely at first that a person come to realize this fact, rather than when bogged down in their normal daily routine. When one realizes that no experience ever benefits or harms our essential nature, this realization allows for much freer, more spontaneous, and less pressurized Qi flow. Having recognized our own essential nature and its inviolability, we can relax and let our minds flow freely in a very natural way. Since the mind and Qi are themselves just the subjective and objective manifestations of a single reality, when the mind flows freely, so does the Qi.

ENDNOTES

1 Lance, James W., M.D., *Migraine and Other Headaches,* Charles Scribner's Sons, NYC, 1986, p. 5

2 Sacks, Oliver W., *Migraine, The Evolution of a Common Disorder,* University of California Press, Berkeley, 1970, p. 151

3 Lance, op.cit., p. 5

4 Ibid., p. 5

5 Wilkinson, Marcia, M.D., *Migraines & Headaches, Understanding, Controlling, and Avoiding the Pain,* Arco Publishing, NYC, 1982, p. 22

6 Sacks, op.cit., p. 152

7 Lance, op.cit., p. 124

8 Ibid., p. 123

9 Sacks, op.cit., p. 119

10 Dudley, Rosemary & Rowland, Wade, *How to Find Relief from Migraine*, Beaufort Books Inc., NYC/Toronto, 1982, p. 153

11 Sacks, op.cit., p. 153

12 Ibid., p. 71

13 Dudley & Rowland, op.cit., p. 32-33

14 Sacks, op.cit., p. 53

15 Ibid., p. 61

16 Ibid., p. 121

17 Ibid., p. 123

18 Rose, F. Clifford & Gavel, M., *Migraine, The Facts*, Oxford Univ. Press, NYC, 1979, p. 10

19 Ibid., p. 10

20 Lance, op.cit., p. 41

21 Sacks, op.cit., p. 54-71

22 Ibid., p. 56

23 Lance, op.cit., p. 47

24 Ibid., p. 47

25 Dudley & Rowland, op.cit., p. 19

26 Sacks, op.cit., p. 68-69

27 Ibid., p. 144

28 Lance, op.cit., p. 38

29 Sacks, op.cit., p. 92

30 Ibid., p. 92

31 Lance, op.cit., p. 39

32 Ibid., p. 39

33 Sacks, op.cit., p. 128

34 Ibid., p. 48

35 Ibid., p. 89

36 Ibid., p. 128

37 Ibid., p. 51

38 Ibid., p. 51

39 Wilkinson, op.cit., p. 16

40 Sacks, op.cit., p.55

41 Ibid., p. 143

42 Rose & Gavel, op.cit., p. 44

43 Wilkinson, op.cit., p. 16

44 Lance, op.cit., p. 35

45 Sacks, op.cit., p. 153-154

46 Evans, Peter, *Mastering Your Migraine,* E.P. Dutton, NYC, 1979, p.27

47 Sacks, op.cit., p 61

48 Evans, op.cit., p. 27

49 Sacks, op.cit., p. 61

50 Lance, op.cit., p. 46

51 Rose & Gavel, op.cit., p. 22

52 Ibid., p. 38

53 Sacks, op.cit., p. 159

54 Ibid., p. 160

55 Ibid., p. 180

56 Ibid., p. 239

57 Ibid., p. 245

58 Dudley & Rowland, op.cit., p. 62

59 Ibid., p. 27

60 Low, Rodolfo, *Migraine, The Breakthrough Study That Explains What Causes It and How It Can Be Completely Prevented Through Diet,* Henry Holt & Co., NYC, 1987

61 Evans, op.cit., p.53-54

62 Rose & Gavel, op.cit., p. 40

63 Ibid., p. 41

64 Lance, op.cit., p. 59

65 Sacks, op.cit., p. 26

66 Ibid., p. 109

67 Ibid., p.90

68 Ibid., p. 109

69 Dudley & Rowland, op.cit., p. 30-31

70 Lance, op.cit., p. 7

71 Rose & Gavel, op.cit., p. 20

72 Lance, op.cit., p. 6

73 Sacks, Oliver W., *Migraine, Understanding a Common Disorder*, Univ. of CA Press, Berkeley, 1985, p. 227

74 Rose & Gavel, op.cit., p. 78

75 Long, James W., M.D., *The Essential Guide to Prescription Drugs*, Harper & Row, NYC, 1985, p. 323

76 Evans, op.cit., p. 82

77 Long, op.cit., p. 512

78 Evans, op.cit., p. 87

79 Long, op.cit., p. 710

80 Ibid., p. 204

81 Sacks, *Understanding...*, op.cit., p. 221-222

82 Ibid., p. 231

83 Ibid., p. 230

84 Ibid., p. 223

85 Ibid., p. 230

86 Sacks, *Evolution...*, op.cit., p. 29

87 Ibid., p. 27

88 Sacks, *Understanding...*, op.cit., p. 231

89 Ibid., p. 232

90 Whether or not the visual displays are real or not is a complex epistemological question. We, as clinicians, tend to dismiss them as

subjectively produced phenomena,a but that dismisal may itself lack depth of perception. Both with psychedelic drugs and in meditative, altered states of consciousness I have "seen" things similar to Hildegaard of Bingen's vision which were absolutely real to me. At those times, my impression was that such visions are always available to us, yet normally we are not receptive to them.

91 Sacks, *Evolution...,* op.cit., p. 160

92 Flaws, Bob, & Wolfe, Honora Lee, *Prince Wen Hui's Cook, Chinese Dietary Therapy*, Paradigm Publications, Brookline, MA, 1984

93 *Time Magazine*, NYC, March 13, 1989, p.51-52

94 Moll, Lucy, "Playing God, When Medicine Plays Monopoly", originally printed in *Vegetarian Times* but quoted in *Nexus*, Boulder, CO, #3, Spring, 1989, p. 42

95 Kukiena, G., "Acupuncture in the Treatment of Migraine", *Fortschritte Der Medezin*, Vol. 103, #25, July 4, 1985, p. 669-672

96 Batra, Y.K., "Acupuncture in the Treatment of Migraine". *American Journal of Acupuncture,* Vol. 14, #2, June, 1986, p. 135-137

97 Junnila, Sappo Y.T., "Acupuncture for Long-term Treatment of Headache in a National Health Center," *American Journal of Acupuncture*, Vol. 14, #4, Dec. 1986, p. 351-353

98 Lenhard, L. & Waite, P.M.E., "Acupuncture in the Prophylactic Treatment of Migraine Headache: A Pilot Study", *New Zealand Medical Journal*, Vol. 96, #738, 1983, p. 663-666

99 Gan Zhen-yuan et al., "Treatment of 31 Cases of Migraine by Penetrating Xuan Lu, Tai Yang Towards Shuai Gu." *Chinese Acupuncture & Moxibustion,* Vol. 3, #4, August 1983, p. 12

100 Loh, L., Nathan, P.W., Schott, G.D., Zilkha, K.J., " Acupuncture Vs. Medical Treatment for Migraine and Muscle Tension Headache," *Journal of Neurology, Neurosurgery, & Psychiatry,* Vol. 47, #4, 1984, p. 333-337

101 Sacks, *Evolution ...,* op.cit., p. 24

102 Ibid., p. 25

103 Ibid., p. 25

104 Long, op.cit., p. 708-713

105 Ibid., p. 202-205

106 Ibid., p. 321-325

107 Ibid., p. 253-256

108 Ibid., p. 626-630

109 Sacks, *Understanding ...*, op.cit., p. 226

110 Long, op.cit., p. 511-514

111 Ibid., p. 120-124

112 Ibid., p. 75-81

ABOUT THE AUTHOR

Bob Flaws, DOM, CMT, Dipl.Ac., is an internationally known practitioner of and author on traditional Chinese medicine. He has written, translated, and edited over fifteen books on various aspects of Oriental medicine and scores of articles by Dr. Flaws have appeared in professional journals both in America and abroad. In addition, Dr. Flaws regularly lectures at many of the major American colleges of acupuncture and Oriental medicine and has been an invited speaker at several national and international medical conferences. His other credits include founding Blue Poppy Press and Blue Poppy Enterprises.

Dr. Flaws originally studied acupuncture with Dr. Tao Xi-yu and at the Shanghai College of Traditional Chinese Medicine where he also studied Chinese herbal medicine and Tuina Chinese remedial massage. He is a founding member and past member of the Board of Directors of the Acupuncture Association of Colorado, a member of the American Association of Acupuncture and Oriental Medicine, was appointed a Research Associate of the Tibetan Medical Society, and is a graduate of the Boulder School of Massage Therapy. Since 1980, Dr. Flaws has conducted a private practice in traditional Chinese medicine in Boulder, CO.

OTHER BOOKS ON CHINESE MEDICINE AVAILABLE FROM BLUE POPPY PRESS

THE BREAST CONNECTION: A Laywoman's Guide to the Treatment of Breast Disease by Chinese Medicine
by Honora Lee Wolfe ISBN 0-936185-13-9 $8.95

NINE OUNCES: A Nine Part Program For The Prevention of AIDS in HIV Positive Persons by Bob Flaws ISBN 0-936185-12-0 $8.95

THE TREATMENT OF CANCER BY INTEGRATED CHINESE-WESTERN MEDICINE by Zhang Dai-zhao, trans. by Zhang Ting-liang & Bob Flaws, ISBN 0-936185-11-2 $16.95

BLUE POPPY ESSAYS: 1988 Translations and Ruminations on Chinese Medicine by Bob Flaws, et al, ISBN 0-936185-10-4 $18.95

A HANDBOOK OF TRADITIONAL CHINESE DERMATOLOGY by Liang Jian-hui, trans. by Zhang Ting-liang & Bob Flaws, ISBN 0-936185-07-4 $14.95

SECRET SHAOLIN FORMULAE FOR THE TREATMENT OF EXTERNAL INJURY by Patriarch De Chan, trans. by Zhang Ting-liang & Bob Flaws, ISBN 0-936185-08-2 $12.95

A HANDBOOK OF TRADITIONAL CHINESE GYNECOLOGY by Zhejiang College of TCM, trans. by Zhang Ting-liang, ISBN 0-936185-06-6 $17.95

FREE & EASY: Traditional Chinese Gynecology for American Women by Bob Flaws, ISBN 0-936185-05-8 $15.95

PRINCE WEN HUI'S COOK: Chinese Dietary Therapy by Bob Flaws & Honora Lee Wolfe, ISBN 0-912111-05-4, $12.95

TURTLE TAIL & OTHER TENDER MERCIES: Traditional Chinese Pediatrics by Bob Flaws ISBN 0-936185-00-7 $14.95

ENDOMETRIOSIS & INFERTILITY AND TRADITIONAL CHINESE MEDICINE: A Laywoman's Guide by Bob Flaws ISBN 0-936185-14-7 $9.95

CLASSICAL MOXIBUSTION SKILLS IN CONTEMPORARY CLINICAL PRACTICE by Sung Baek ISBN 0-936185-16-3 $10.95